Perimenopause *the* Natural Way

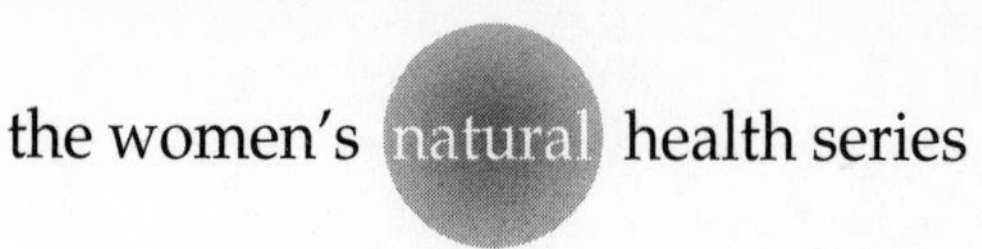

Perimenopause *the* Natural Way

Deborah Gordon, M.D., Series Editor

Keralyn Brenner

and

Deborah Gordon, M.D.

A Lynn Sonberg Book

John Wiley & Sons, Inc.
New York • Chichester • Weinheim • Brisbane • Singapore • Toronto

Published by John Wiley & Sons, Inc.
Published simultaneously in Canada

Illustrations by Jackie Aher

Design and production by Navta Associates, Inc.

Library of Congress Cataloging-in-Publication Data

Gordon, Deborah (Deborah R.)
Perimenopause the natural way / Keralyn Brenner, Deborah Gordon.
p. cm. — (The women's natural health series)
Includes index.
ISBN 0-471-37960-3 (pbk.)
1. Perimenopause—Complications—Alternative treatment.
I. Brenner, Keralyn. II. Title. III. Series.

RG186 .G66 2000
618.1'75—dc21 00-035907

Printed in the United States of America

10 9 8 7 6 5 4 3 2 1

Important Note

This book is for informational purposes only. It is not intended to take the place of medical advice from a trained medical professional. Readers are advised to consult a physician or other qualified health professional regarding treatment of all of their health problems or before acting on any of the information or advice in this book.

This book is intended to provide selected information about perimenopause. Research about perimenopause is ongoing and subject to conflicting interpretations. As a result, there is no guarantee that what we know about this subject won't change with time.

Contents

Perimenopause *the* Natural Way

Introduction

By Deborah Gordon, M.D.

You're only in your mid-30s and you absolutely do not want to hear the word *menopause* applied to you, even with the "peri" before it. You're not there yet. You're still young, you're barely where you want to be in life, and you haven't even had the chance to have those kids you've been dreaming about. But you know something just isn't right with your body. You're tired all the time, as well as irritable and anxious. Your breasts are sore and tender, and you've started to have irregular periods. Some of your friends and colleagues feel this way too.

You wonder what's going on. You're experiencing perimenopause, the transitional years before menopause, when you will stop menstruating completely. Perimenopause can last for 10 years. It doesn't mean you've lost your fertility, your youth, or your health. Yet if you're experiencing uncomfortable symptoms, your hormones are out of balance. This book will teach you how to regain the balance in both your physical health and emotional well-being.

In recent years, more and more people have been turning to alternative or complementary medicine for answers to their health problems. Although a small percentage of Americans have long sought out holistic practitioners, recent years have witnessed a phenomenal explosion in the use of herbal remedies, acupuncture, homeopathy, chiropractic medicine, mind/body medicine, and a host of other alternative therapies. These approaches are no longer experimental options to conventional medicine but rather they are well-respected and well-researched treatment modalities that enhance health. Complementary medicine is now widely used for everything from colds and flus to chronic fatigue syndrome to hypertension.

If you are experiencing uncomfortable or troubling perimenopausal symptoms, there are many compelling reasons to explore alternative healing. First and foremost, based on the clinical experience of hundreds of practitioners in the United States, these techniques can help you reverse your symptoms. This is not to say that alternative health care offers miracles, but your symptoms are caused by a multitude of chronic factors, and many of these respond to natural remedies. For example, hormonal imbalance is one of the main culprits in your discomfort. By altering diet, taking nutritional supplements, using herbs, and practicing relaxation exercises, many women are able to restore hormonal balance.

In addition to reversing your symptoms, alternative treatments will also enhance your overall health. Indeed, these two outcomes are closely linked—that is, in general, the better your health, the less likely you are to experience perimenopausal symptoms. By exercising regularly, eating healthy, and using natural remedies, you will enjoy a higher level of physical vitality.

As we'll discuss later in this book, alternative therapies can also give you more control over this often difficult time of life. While health care practitioners play an essential role in natural medicine, self-care is just as important. By forming a positive partnership with your practitioner based on mutual respect and responsibility, you can face the challenges of perimenopause with greater confidence and less anxiety.

This book offers an individualized approach for making it

through perimenopause. If you're serious about improving your health, the program described here will provide an excellent start. You can follow it, or you can pick and choose the methods of healing to which you're most drawn, and chart your progress. You'll find that natural methods for reversing symptoms will give you the widest range for experimenting, as well as many opportunities to improve your health.

As a family physician practicing both conventional and complementary forms of medicine, I have seen patients make incredible improvements in their health through holistic therapies. By changing their diet, exercising regularly, using herbs and nutritional supplements, and decreasing stress, they have regained their vitality, which in turn has allowed them to glide through perimenopause with ease.

Perimenopause is an ideal time to look inward and to take the steps necessary to enhance your physical and emotional well-being. You will also be laying the foundation for continued good health and a new understanding of yourself and your body.

CHAPTER ONE

What Is Perimenopause?

Perimenopause is the phase of a woman's life leading up to menopause during which her levels of reproductive hormones begin to fluctuate. (Menopause officially begins only after you have not menstruated for 12 consecutive months.) Perimenopause can result in wide-ranging symptoms that include anxiety, irritability, memory lapses, and breast tenderness. Many hormonal problems that are commonly described as menopausal actually belong to this preceding transitional phase.

If you feel you are in perimenopause, pay attention to what you are experiencing and respect the changes your body is going through. In fact, you can become your own best authority on what is happening to your reproductive system. This takes some quiet thought and listening to your inner self. Remember, perimenopause is a time, not a problem, so treat yourself accordingly. You may notice irregular periods; changes in normal mood patterns, sleep, or sexual drive; unexplained weight gain or food cravings; even new patterns of digestion or headaches.

These symptoms are all clues to the hormonal fluctuations of perimenopause.

If this sounds like what you are experiencing, you are not alone. More than 20 million American women are now in this phase of life, reflecting the aging of the populous baby-boomer generation. Although the American medical establishment had begun to recognize the differing symptoms of perimenopause in the 1970s, the majority of physicians had not heard of perimenopause before the 1990s, when menopause began to receive attention in the press. Most medical schools still don't include perimenopause discussions in classes and some doctors dismiss symptoms as being psychologically based.

The more you know about perimenopause, the more able you will be to take care of yourself as your body adjusts to changes in hormone status. Being informed about the physiological changes that are occurring, the symptoms to watch for, and the various means of preventing and treating them can give you a lot of control over how you feel during this phase of your reproductive life. By identifying symptoms such as foggy memory or feeling blue, you can take action and make lifestyle changes, such as eating better and exercising more, that can ease these annoyances. Taking the mystery out of perimenopause can also reduce worries and stress, which themselves can bring on symptoms. And by being more informed, you will be a better patient who can communicate valuable information if you decide you need to consult a physician.

When Does Perimenopause Begin?

The changes in hormone production characteristic of perimenopause can take place over a period of 10 to 13 years, until menopause arrives. The average age of women who begin perimenopause is 47, but some women experience these changes as early as their late 30s. Other women enter perimenopause in their 50s. The timing can vary widely from woman to woman, and each experience can still be considered normal. Not all women experience negative symptoms during perimenopause, but for the women who do, these symptoms are very real and very unpleasant. Learning how to manage symptoms will help you make this transition with more confidence and less stress.

The Menstrual Cycle and Perimenopausal Changes

To give you an idea of what occurs within your body as perimenopausal changes begin to surface, let's first take a look at the normal menstrual cycle that is typical of a woman's reproductive years. This cycle is regulated by hormones. During the month, in response to hormones produced by the brain's pituitary gland—follicle-stimulating hormone (FSH) and luteinizing hormone (LH)—the uterus thickens, preparing to receive a fertilized egg. If a woman does not become pregnant, the thickened lining of the uterus sloughs off and menstrual bleeding results.

The ovaries, which are located within a woman's pelvis, contain egg follicles—eggs that are unfertilized and inactive. FSH and LH stimulate the follicles to ripen. One of the follicles grows into a mature egg, which will eventually make its way down the fallopian tubes that lead to the uterus, and will possibly be fertilized by the male sperm. While the follicles ripen, they also begin to produce estrogen and progesterone. Estrogen production dominates in the first half of the menstrual cycle, peaking at mid-month when ovulation occurs. Progesterone production dominates in the second 2 weeks of the menstrual cycle leading up to menstruation.

At birth, a woman's ovaries contain as many as 400,000 eggs. By the time she approaches menopause, her supply of eggs has greatly diminished. Estrogen and progesterone produced by

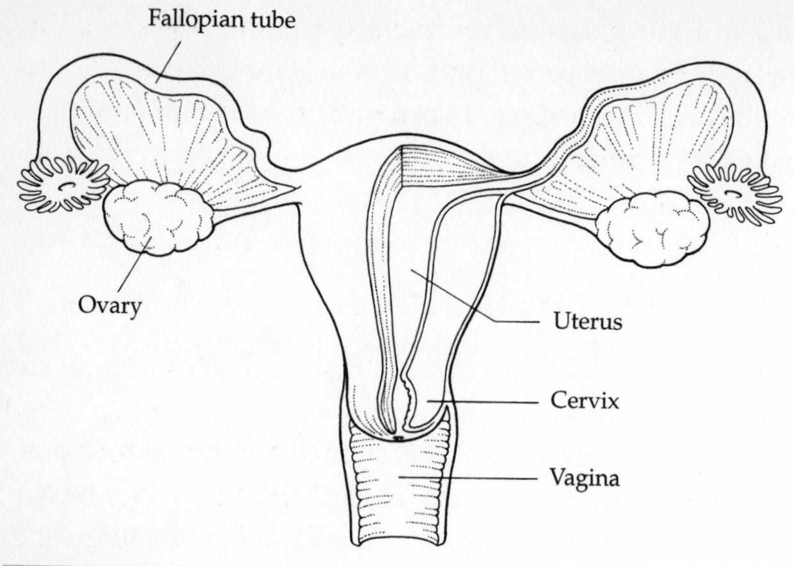

Female reproductive organs

the follicles in the ovaries decline as well. In response, the pituitary gland begins to produce higher and higher levels of FSH and LH to stimulate estrogen and progesterone production, which are produced in great quantity. FSH levels can rise as much as 10-fold and LH levels can rise 4-fold. The end result of perimenopause is that various reproduction hormones no longer work together with precise timing.

TESTING FOR PERIMENOPAUSE

Any time during a woman's first 6 days of her period, a blood test is taken to measure FSH in units called milli-international units per milliliter. Clinicians look for a reading above 30 to indicate overproduction of FSH, indicating that the patient is in perimenopause. However, this test is not always reliable. Taken during a month when a woman's period is normal, the test will yield no sign of abnormal hormone production. To confirm a diagnosis of perimenopause, the test should be repeated the following month as well. One drawback is that this lab work is expensive. Informed observation of symptoms can be just as telling.

Your Hormones: A Balancing Act

Hormones are the chemicals that regulate most of the body's internal functions, including body temperature, digestion, sexual development and reproduction, perimenopause, and eventually menopause. Hormone function is controlled by the reproductive endocrine system, a collection of glands that produce hormones. These hormones are secreted into the bloodstream, which carries them to their respective destinations throughout the body. The endocrine system is so complex that some hormones serve only to stimulate certain glands, which in turn produce other hormones.

The two primary female hormones are estrogen and progesterone, both of which are produced by the ovaries. At puberty the body's estrogen levels increase to enhance the growth of secondary sex characteristics, such as breast development and widening hips. Estrogen also stimulates the hypothalamus gland, which is located at the base of the brain. This is where the body produces gonadotropin-releasing hormone (GnRH). The secretion of GnRH begins the process of ovulation.

All of the key reproductive hormones—estrogen, progesterone, GnRH, FSH, and LH—must be in sync with one another. If the balance is thrown off even slightly, your body reacts by manifesting symptoms. The purpose of this book is to teach you how to help your body to balance and regulate your hormones so that you will not experience a wide range of unpleasant symptoms.

Hormone Peaks and Valleys

The previous description of how hormone production changes during perimenopause paints a simple picture. But hormone production does not actually decline as smoothly as suggested. During a woman's normal menstrual cycle, events take place that are directed by various hormones acting in concert in a coordinated and well-timed sequence. But with perimenopause, it is as if the hormones that are partners in this dance miss a few steps. One partner stumbles and another speeds up. The dancers try new steps.

Estrogen levels in the first few days of a woman's cycle can peak, rising 1000%, and then they can plummet. In one study, conducted in 1996 at the University of Washington, a group of 300 women, ages 40 to 45, were found to have estrogen levels comparable to women in their 20s. However, during the first part of their menstrual cycle, they had estrogen levels higher than the younger women.

Look for the Signs

The most obvious sign of perimenopause is an irregular menstrual cycle. Your period may occur more frequently or not as often. Menstrual flow might be exceptionally heavy or light. Some women in perimenopause have hot flashes and night sweats. Dry skin and hair, a decreased interest in sex, and thinning and drying of vaginal walls are also possibilities.

One theory of the origin of perimenopausal complaints is that *fluctuations* in estrogen levels—not high or low levels of estrogen per se—trigger symptoms. High estrogen levels can trigger hot flashes as well as typical PMS-like (premenstrual syndrome) symptoms such as irritability and anxiety. Low estrogen is associated in some women with mood swings and problems with short-term memory.

Symptoms of perimenopause may also be triggered by low levels of progesterone. Since this hormone normally stabilizes the uterine lining and signals when to slough it off, a lack of progesterone can cause you to skip a period. Low progesterone can also lead to "the blues." FSH can play a role in perimenopausal problems, possibly triggering hot flashes and night sweats. FSH can indirectly cause blood vessels that lie just beneath the skin to dilate. If this occurs, you may feel unexpectedly warm.

Redefining "Normal"

It is important to remember that there is not just one "normal" type of perimenopause or one typical pattern of menstruation. Just about any sequence of events is possible because several hormones play a role in triggering perimenopausal symptoms. Some women stop their period for a whole year and then begin having regular periods again. Others have periods every 3 weeks or even every 10 days and then skip a month. And some women pass through this phase of life with few, if any, symptoms.

Your personal experience with perimenopause depends on many factors, ranging from your social situation to other health conditions Women in cultures where age is more revered show less problems during both the perimenopausal and menopausal years. A key factor in which you have great influence is in choosing the quality of the foods you eat, how much you exercise, and how you feel about your body and the changes it is going through.

Everyone is different in terms of their medical history and how they take care of themselves. Consider Carla, age 49, who for years was plagued by migraine headaches and was very prone to PMS. As her period started to become irregular, her headaches became more frequent, were of longer duration, and were more painful. She also had more weepy spells and was bothered by bloating. Carla tried many treatments including Chinese herbs and a change to a healthful diet. She had been subsisting on nutrient-poor refined and processed foods and switched to eating more natural ingredients. In particular, she vowed to stay away from refined sugar and caffeine. To her delight, her mood swings began to stabilize, but her headaches continued to come and go for some time until her body stabilized from the dietary changes.

And there are women who don't recall having any symptoms of perimenopause. Emma, who is now in her 70s, likes to tell the story of her one and only hot flash. She was giving a talk before a group of people and felt her cheeks redden and perspiration start to form. Emma recalls the embarrassment, which was compounded by the fear of not knowing what it was.

Why are some women more successful than others in treating symptoms? And why do some women glide through this transition, while others have such a difficult time? Individual biochemistry is the answer you'll get from most doctors and practitioners, but that's only the tip of the iceberg. As you'll learn in this book, environmental factors, hormonal imbalances, poor diet, life stresses, inactivity, and many other factors *that are all within your control* can influence how easy (or difficult) this time will be for you.

Attending to Your Needs

Now is a good time to get in touch with your body. It's important to identify what's occurring so that you can receive appropriate medical advice if needed. If you don't tell your physician you suspect you're in perimenopause, you may be prescribed tranquilizers for your anxiety, sleeping pills for your sleeping problems, and antidepressants for your mood swings while your underlying hormonal imbalances are ignored.

The following chapters give you the tools for shepherding yourself through your version of perimenopause. Chapter 2 tells you more about the physical and emotional symptoms of perimenopause you may experience and their origins. You are given an overview of the program and the tools for creating your own personal perimenopause journal. Use your journal to track your symptoms and follow the progress of the treatments you choose.

This book will also guide you through a six-step transitional program that includes information on cleansing the liver, using natural progesterone, following dietary recommendations, using nutritional and herbal medicine to balance hormones, benefiting from exercise and mind/body therapies, and addressing emotional issues.

Treat yourself to these ways of managing this time of transition. The recommendations given in this book have been useful for many women, and are likely to ease your passage through perimenopause as well.

CHAPTER TWO

The Cycle of Change: Signs of Perimenopause

How will you know that you're in perimenopause? Your body will begin to give you signs. Probably the most noticeable first sign will be that your menstrual cycle will begin to become irregular. If your cycles have always been irregular, you'll notice some change from this irregularity. You may have an unusually heavy menstrual flow, which is called menorrhagia, or you may experience an especially light flow or spotting.

Changing patterns of hormone production trigger these menstrual variations and can bring on related annoyances including insomnia, anxiety, night sweats, mood swings, and headaches. Diminished hormone levels can also cause memory problems, concentration difficulties, and a decreased interest in sex. These later complaints can continue into menopause as well.

This chapter explains the common signs of perimenopause. Medical problems that can induce and worsen symptoms are also presented, including uterine fibroids, endometriosis, thyroid problems, and overtaxed adrenals.

It may seem as though the signs of perimenopause and the causes of various related discomforts indicate a disease or a condition to be treated and even resisted. Yet it's important to know that perimenopause is a transitional period that you will adapt to, not conquer. It is not a malfunction but an adjustment. By seeking to understand the changes your body is undergoing, your mind will have a stronger foundation for assisting you in making this adaptation comfortably and wisely.

Perimenopause is a natural part of a woman's life cycle, as normal and expected as menstruation and pregnancy. If you recognize this, you are more likely to have an easier passage through this period. Minor discomforts can more easily be taken in stride as you give your body credit for working its way toward this completion of your reproductive years. Listen to your body. Do you need more nourishing food and more rest? Make sure you get them. Your body is busy replacing old chemical pathways with new ones designed to keep you moving forward for many more years. A cycle of your life is ending, but a new one is being born.

Take comfort in the truth that you won't necessarily be troubled by every symptom described. Perimenopause is a highly individual experience. The probability of whether you experiencing one symptom or another depends on the general condition of your health as these changes begin. Diet, exercise, whether you smoke, alcohol consumption, history of reproductive problems, and the amount of stress you have in your life can all make a difference—as can individual biochemistry and genetic background, over which you have no control.

Why Your Symptoms May Seem Different

Many factors determine your journey through perimenopause. Some are controllable by you and others are not.

Diet is definitely related to symptoms. Women who consume more fruits and vegetables and less processed foods generally have an easier time in perimenopause. Phytoestrogenic foods (discussed in Chapter 6) balance hormones. Meat and meat products wreak havoc on your hormones and organs.

Stress can also influence symptoms. Do you keep a busy schedule, either at work or balancing family demands? In fact, studies have shown that busy women in urban environments experience greater discomfort from perimenopausal symptoms than their rural counterparts. As we'll explain later in this book, stress not only causes and intensifies symptoms, but it affects your overall health and well-being.

If your experience seems to put you in the "high-risk" category for symptoms, don't worry. Your willingness to make some lifestyle changes gives you a distinct advantage for making it through perimenopause symptom-free.

Irregular Periods

Women are cyclical beings, the reproductive functions of the body rhythmically repeating as naturally as the moon passes through its cycle and the tides rise and fall. The menstrual cycle occurs once every month, about every 28 days. But for some women, the cycle can be several days shorter or several days longer and can still be considered normal. Menstrual flow usually lasts 3 to 5 days. However, some women in good health regularly menstruate only 2 days, whereas other equally healthy women have periods that can last as long as a week.

In the normal menstrual cycle, one of the little sacs (follicles) within the ovaries releases an egg, or ovulates. This follicle then secretes progesterone, a hormone which, along with estrogen, thickens the uterine lining, increases the number of blood vessels within the uterine tissues, and prepares the uterus to nurture the egg once it has been fertilized. But if the egg is not fertilized, the follicle begins to disintegrate and progesterone production declines. The lining of the uterus also begins to break down and then slough off, a process you experience as menstruation.

As you pass through perimenopause, your periods may become quite irregular. With unstable hormone levels that occur during perimenopause, some ovarian follicles may no longer function. Consequently, ovulation is infrequent or sporadic and insufficient progesterone is produced. Your period may skip a month or come more frequently. Such irregularity can be an annoyance. You may be accustomed to planning your business travel and even your personal life around the days you expect to begin menstruating. You may feel irritable and not realize why you are feeling particularly sensitive. Fortunately, specific foods and herbs can help regulate the menstrual cycle. Supplemental hormones can also be effective and will be described in Chapter 5.

Heavy Bleeding

Your menstrual irregularity may be accompanied by heavy bleeding, known by the medical term *menorrhagia*. There may be rapid, heavy flow over a brief amount of time, or more moderate flow over many days. During perimenopause, it is not uncommon for women to have periods that last 7 to 10 days. Besides being inconvenient, heavy bleeding can also lead to anemia. Elevated estrogen levels, when combined with lowered progesterone levels, can lead to menorrhagia. Women who are overweight, smoke, or overindulge in alcohol are at higher risk of having elevated estrogen levels. A diet low in nutrients such as vitamin C and bioflavonoids can also lead to heavy flow. Various medical conditions, discussed next, are also associated with excessive bleeding.

Fibroids

These benign growths of muscle and connective tissue are known by the medical term *myomas*. They are usually located in the wall of the uterus. About 40% of ovulating women have fibroids, which become more common as perimenopause approaches. Fibroids can also cause menorrhagia.

Fibroids are stimulated by estrogen and can increase in size until they begin to place pressure on neighboring anatomy such as the bowel and bladder. Often, hysterectomy is recommended to remove these growths. However, at menopause, when estrogen production dramatically declines, fibroids will naturally shrink. Following a low-fat diet, supplementing with certain nutrients and herbs, and avoiding excessive stress can also help prevent and treat fibroids. Persistent fibroids may need medical attention if they cause excessive bleeding or physical discomfort.

Endometriosis

In this serious medical condition, cells that make up the lining of the uterus break away and migrate outside the uterine cavity to nearby areas such as the cervix and bowel. Less frequently, they also travel to many other parts of the body. These cells continue to respond to hormones as if they were still part of the uterus and can cause bleeding wherever they are. A significant number of women with endometriosis have heavy menstrual bleeding. There are many ways to address this problem without resorting to surgery or prescription hormones. These self-care options will be discussed in Chapters 5 and 7. Additionally, practitioners of acupuncture and homeopathy can offer less invasive methods of treatment.

Hot Flashes

Estrogen levels do not necessarily decline gradually during perimenopause. They can plummet and then soar and drop again within a single cycle. Low estrogen during the first 2 weeks of the menstrual cycle, when estrogen production is slowly increasing, can trigger hot flashes. About 30% of women in their 40s experience these before the onset of menopause. If you have a hot flash, you will most likely feel unusually warm in the face and neck. You may also feel heat in your upper chest area. It is not the deep tissues of your body that have become hot; if you measured your body temperature with a thermometer, you would not find that you have a temperature as you might if you were sick. Rather, when a hot flash occurs, it is your skin temperature that suddenly elevates. The skin may flush and redden. Frequency of hot flashes can vary greatly. Having just a few hot flashes a day is typical. Most hot flashes last from 3 to 5 minutes but can be as short as a few seconds. A hot flash can bring on perspiration, the body's attempt to cool itself. As the perspiration evaporates, you will probably feel chilled. If you have a series of hot flashes, you may find yourself putting on and taking off your jacket all day long. Dressing lightly and layering clothing is definitely the fashion recommendation if you are troubled by hot flashes, but this book will also provide you with ways to reduce or eliminate them altogether!

Hot Flash Chemistry

The hypothalamus helps determine sleep patterns, reaction to stress, mood, sex drive, and metabolic rate, as well as the release of pituitary hormones, suggesting that midlife changes in the hypothalamus may be involved in the onset of other menopause symptoms as well.

It is not yet known what causes the series of events called a hot flash. Estrogen undoubtedly plays a role, since this hormone has an effect on the hypothalamus. This part of the brain functions as a bridge or link between the hormonal or endocrine system and the nervous system. It also stimulates the pituitary gland, which produces follicle-stimulating hormone (FSH) and leuteinizing hormone (LH), to direct ovulation and the output of estrogen and progesterone by the ovaries. The hypothalamus affects the vascular system, altering regional blood flow. Lowered estrogen levels may influence the metabolism of the hormone norepinephrine, the stress hormone produced by the adrenal glands. Norepinephrine affects both the body temperature–regulating function and the relationship between the nervous system and the hormonal system.

Other Symptoms: Anxiety, Irritation, and Heart Palpitations

While flushing is the primary sign of a hot flash, the experience may be accompanied by other annoyances including anxiety, irritation, and even panic. If you are aware that you are in the middle of a hot flash, these annoyances may be easier to ride out. Nonetheless, they are frightening and can affect not only your overall well-being but your day-to-day life. Diet and nutritional and herbal supplementation can effectively control these symptoms.

Heart palpitations can occur secondary to hot flashes. However, if heart palpitations occur at times when no hot flash has occurred, you should consult a physician, as palpitations can be a symptom of more serious medical conditions.

Night Sweats

Hot flashes at night are called night sweats. These can be intense, and as they disrupt sleep, night sweats can lead to fatigue. If night sweats are particularly frequent, you may be

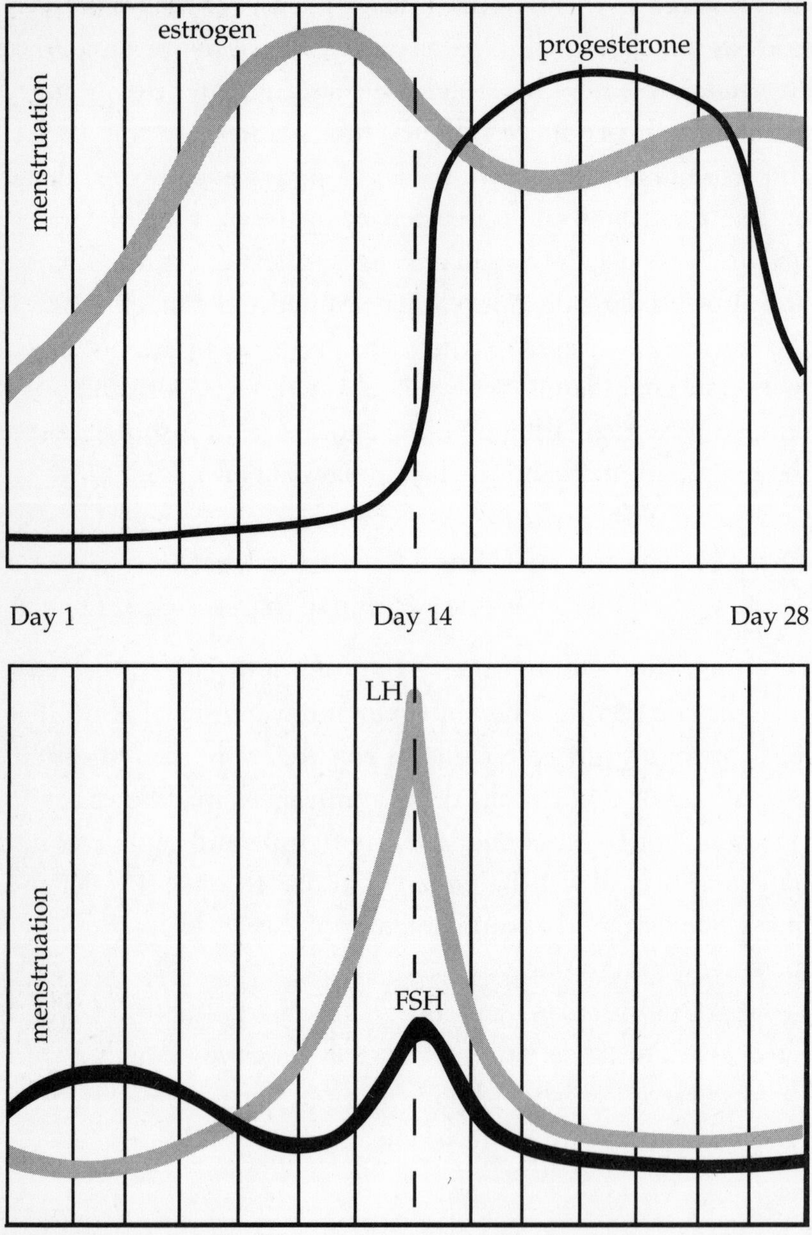

Hormone levels during menstrual cycle (this chart is not exact, but representative of the average menstrual cycle)

deprived of the form of sleep associated with dreaming, which is known as rapid eye movement (REM) sleep. REM deprivation can lead to depression. If night sweats trouble you, be sure to make your bed using several coverlets of different weights so that you can adjust these to suit your body temperature. Many women also find that lowering the room temperature helps.

Fatigue

Feeling tired is one of the most common symptoms of perimenopause. Your body's energy supply is in constant and heavy demand due to basic biological changes and a wide fluctuation of hormone activity. If you're losing sleep because of stress or for other reasons, this can also contribute to fatigue. In fact, studies have shown that the loss of only one night's sleep can result in tiredness, irritability, inability to concentrate, and mood swings. These annoyances are considered symptoms of perimenopause but may be indirectly related.

During this time, you may feel the need to take an occasional afternoon nap. Julie, a retail shoe buyer, began to experience extreme midafternoon fatigue at her job for a major international department store. At first she tried to push through her tiredness. One of her colleagues suggested taking a short nap in the afternoon. Yet because of her exceptionally strong work ethic, she didn't allow herself a moment's rest during the day. However, the fatigue persisted and Julie was forced to take a little quiet time in the afternoon. Surprisingly, a half-hour of quiet time (not necessarily sleep) rejuvenated her enough to finish her day and accomplish her tasks.

In most cases, fatigue will subside as your body adjusts to the peaks and valleys of hormone production. If your fatigue is a by-product of poor diet, however, basic changes will need to be made. See Chapter 6 for more information on dietary recommendations.

Mood Swings

Sex hormones have a profound effect on the function of the central nervous system, and mood swings can be the result. Reduced production of estrogen during the first half of the menstrual cycle can bring on hot flashes, as well as signal the thyroid gland to churn out more FSH, the hormone that stimulates the ovaries to produce more estrogen. FSH levels soar, and consequently estrogen levels double. High levels of estrogen, relative to progesterone, can trigger anxiety and irritability.

In addition, during perimenopause, progesterone levels can drop. Progesterone binds to the same sites in the brain as does gamma-aminobutyric acid (GABA), a neurochemical that dampens anxiety. (Of note is that the popular antidepressant diazepam, commonly known as Valium, also binds to the same sites.) As mentioned previously, hot flashes and night sweats, which disrupt sleep, can also make mood swings more likely. Some women's lives are brought to a halt by these symptoms and they often seek help from physicians and counselors—where help may come in the form of antidepressants if perimenopause is misdiagnosed and underlying conditions aren't addressed. However, the good news is that if you take action to ease one symptom, others are likely to improve as well.

Angry?

During perimenopause little things may just get to you. In fact, things that never bothered you before, such as your partner's inability to get the socks *into* the hamper, may infuriate you. Are you going crazy? No, spontaneous anger—even rage—is a by-product of your fluctuating hormones.

But before you try to mask these feelings or make excuses for them, take a moment and notice why you are acting out. There is some truth in your reaction, even though it may be exaggerated, and this is your chance to find out what really is going on inside of you. Your anger is sending you messages. What may begin as a crisis may become an opportunity. Communicated with love to those nearest you, the sharing of your thoughts has the potential of improving your relationships and increasing intimacy.

Insomnia

Can't sleep? For the women who begin to suffer through sleepless nights at the outset of perimenopause, life quickly becomes unbearable. Without a good night's sleep (or several), you are not able to continue living at your normal pace and other symptoms you may be experiencing will seem exacerbated by your fatigue.

Fortunately, there are several easy ways to combat the insomnia associated with perimenopause, and the easiest one is exercise. More remedies will be discussed throughout the book, as well as the underlying causes of your symptoms.

Memory Lapses and Loss of Concentration

Memory lapses can be one of the most dismaying symptoms of perimenopause. You might be walking into another room to get a needle and thread and find yourself not recalling what you were looking for in the first place. The plot thickens if you play out this scenario working in a hectic office.

With perimenopause, you may experience your brain taking little holidays. Here's what scientists currently believe is going on chemically. Estrogen may affect certain brain enzymes. These in turn may alter the metabolism of acetylcholine, a neurotransmitter thought to be critical for memory function. Estrogen stimulates neurons, the fundamental components of the nervous system that make communication within the body possible, to grow new branches. Estrogen also helps generate new synapses, points between neurons where data travel from one nerve to another. This network of neurons makes it possible for you to learn and remember. During perimenopause, the peaks and valleys of hormonal activity can wreak havoc on your mind.

Research shows that declining estrogen levels affect verbal rather than spatial memory. If you're introduced to people at a party, you may have more difficulty remembering their names. However, you will still be able to remember where you parked your car and the route to take to return home.

Low estrogen levels for some women can cause the feeling of brain fogging. Caffeine no longer does the trick and is ineffective at sharpening your mind. However, giving yourself more nutrient-rich foods, especially those that supply B vitamins and essential fatty acids, can help reverse this tendency. You will also be more alert if you drink plenty of water throughout the day and exercise regularly. These good habits increase blood flow to the brain. See Chapters 6 and 8 for specific recommendations.

SEEING THROUGH BRAIN FOG

There is another way to look at brain fogging. It may be your inner wisdom trying to break through. Thinking that occurs via the left lobe of the brain is linear. The left lobe of the brain is where verbal information is stored. Here you plan your day and manage the details of your life. Men tend to think more frequently in this mode. In contrast, the right lobe of your brain "thinks" without using words and is skilled at scanning the world and taking in a whole picture of events. The right lobe gives you intuitive information. Women excel at this way of thinking.

Perhaps with perimenopause, the brain fogging you are experiencing is really an opening of this more female consciousness. Perimenopause brings some women new and highly useful insights into their own personal world as well as the world at large. In many traditional societies, such as that of Native Americans, tribe members recognized that elder women had special wisdom and respected them as counselors who could help ensure the survival of the tribe. If your thinking becomes clouded and vague, take a moment to consider if some messages are coming through all the same.

Perimenopause and Sexuality

Symptoms associated with perimenopause always include changes that occur to vaginal tissue and sexual drive. Vaginal tissue is made up of many layers of cushioning cells. When estrogen is in adequate supply, these cells remain resilient and strong. But as estrogen levels decline, the outer layers of vaginal mucosal cells, approximately six layers deep, can become thin. As a result, intercourse may become somewhat irritating and even painful.

During perimenopause, production of vaginal fluid begins to fluctuate and decline. A lack of lubrication, coupled with thinning vaginal tissue, can make sexual activity all the more irritating to vaginal walls. Fortunately, many treatments and behavior changes have been proven to alleviate these conditions (see Chapters 5 and 9). Most women can continue to enjoy the sexual aspect of their lives well through perimenopause and menopause and into their later years.

How the Body Changes

As ovarian function wanes, blood flow to the pelvic area declines. In the areas of the vagina and vulva (the outer portion of the female genitalia), this decrease can be as much as 60 percent. Pubic hair also thins and becomes coarser.

The most pronounced changes occur to the vagina. Vaginal tissue is made up of many layers of cushioning cells. When the supply of estrogen is adequate, these cells remain resilient and strong. However, with menopause, the outer layers of vaginal mucosal cells, approximately six layers deep, can become thin. The surface of the vagina begins to flatten and it loses its rough, ridged appearance. The vagina also decreases in depth and the walls of the vagina begin to lose their elasticity as fibrous connective tissue replaces muscle cells. However, orgasmic contractions of the vagina still occur after menopause.

Another result of diminished blood flow is that production of vaginal fluid begins to fluctuate and is less copious. A lack of lubricating fluid can cause intercourse to be somewhat painful and also irritating to vaginal tissue. If this tissue has thinned, sexual activity can be all the more irritating to the vaginal walls. Fortunately, many treatments and behavior changes have been shown to alleviate these conditions. These are covered in subsequent chapters.

Drying Skin

There is no cause for alarm. Drying skin and wrinkles will not show up overnight. However, just as vaginal tissue is changing, your exterior skin tissues begin to alter during the perimenopausal years. The production of collagen, the protein that keeps your skin firm, decreases, which is possibly linked to a reduction in estrogen levels. The skin becomes less elastic and wrinkles can appear. But as there are various ways to slow vaginal aging, the body's exterior tissues also respond well to smart eating choices and a healthy lifestyle. The oil-soluble vitamins, A and E, nourish skin tissue, and vitamin C is critical for the formation of collagen. Essential fatty acids lubricate the skin, and being well hydrated by drinking plenty of water can restore volume to skin tissue and dispel fine wrinkles. Avoiding smoking, which can dry skin tissue, can also significantly improve your appearance, while adding years and quality to your life.

Hypothyroidism: Symptoms That Masquerade as Perimenopause

Symptoms such as memory loss, irritability, and heavy menstrual flow, automatically attributed to perimenopause, may in fact be due to a thyroid gland that is functioning sluggishly. This butterfly-shaped gland, part of the body's endocrine system, is located in the neck just above the Adam's apple. The most well-known function of the thyroid gland is metabolic regulation—that is, the rate at which food is converted to energy. But the thyroid also influences the regulation of body temperature and heart rate, and along with the adrenal glands, the rate at which carbohydrates are turned into fuel.

Because the thyroid gland impacts various body functions, when thyroid function slows, as it typically does in women in their 40s and 50s, various complaints can result. Besides those already mentioned, you may experience muscle stiffness and general fatigue, headaches, depression, a tendency to feel chilly, poor appetite, and, at the same time, weight gain.

If you are experiencing any of these symptoms, you should be tested for hypothyroidism. You can ask your physician to give you the standard blood test that assesses thyroid function. It measures the two types of the thyroid hormone thyroxine: T3 and T4, as well as the messenger hormone, TSH (thyroid-stimulating hormone). However, this standard test is often not sensitive enough to reveal mild cases of hypothyroidism, which can still cause problems.

Being better informed about your thyroid function can help you avoid a misdiagnosis of your condition. If hypothyroidism is causing you to be depressed, you don't need an antidepressant. If a sluggish thyroid is causing headaches, although you may need immediate help for the pain, you will want to treat the underlying cause.

Now that you have some idea of the various body changes that occur during the perimenopause years, get ready to get in touch with how you are feeling. In the following chapter, you will learn the six steps of the program, and you will be given the opportunity to create your own personal perimenopause journal.

CHAPTER THREE

Balance Your Hormones, Balance Your Life: Getting Started on the Six-Step Transitional Program

Now that you have a greater understanding of your own symptoms, you're well on your way to managing this transition. Each woman's program will vary depending on her own symptoms and needs, and you'll be pleased with the results you gain from creating your journal and your individualized version of the six-step program outlined in this chapter.

It's never too early—or too late—to get started. You can begin by reading this chapter carefully to get an overview of the six-step program that will be detailed in the following chapters. By following this plan, you will benefit by:

- Improving your overall feelings of health and well-being
- Learning to prevent, manage, or even reverse your perimenopausal symptoms

- Reducing the likelihood of menopause-related health conditions later in life, such as heart disease and osteoporosis
- Controlling stress and anxiety
- Preparing your body, mind, and spirit for the perimenopausal transition
- Creating balance in your life

Preparing Your Mind

It used to be that, for most doctors, health was simply a matter of body parts functioning properly. When they didn't, the mighty arsenal of medications was called on to repair the problem. If those failed to work, even more aggressive action in the form of surgery was pursued.

Certainly drugs and surgical procedures are often necessary to cure illness and injury. But today we've learned that the mind, as well as the spirit, can play a pivotal role in the healing process.

In Eastern societies, as well as indigenous cultures in the West, the link between physical and mental well-being has always been clear. Meditation, religion, hypnosis, and yoga can all play a key role in maintaining or restoring health.

Until recently, this integrationist approach was largely ridiculed by physicians as primitive superstition. Yet growing scientific and public interest has led to the rapid evolution of a new field: mind/body medicine.

Working with studies demonstrating the relationship between physical health and such variables as mood, attitude, and spirituality, pioneering researchers are now expanding the boundaries of medical science. Do people with a positive attitude stand a better chance of recovering from sickness? Can depression weaken the immune system, leading to physical illness? What contributions can meditation and relaxation therapies make to the healing process? Many, and they are important, which is why we focus on the mind and spirit—as well as the body—during perimenopause.

Finding the Balance Within

Before you can adapt to your hormones, you may want to first look at the pace your life has taken. Many women today simply do too much, too often, and without the help or recognition they need and deserve. In today's society, kids' and partners' needs often come first and women find that the greatest imbalance they face comes from overwork. Often, that very first hot flash or memory blip brings with it a close examination of life and its purpose. You can use this to your advantage.

Balancing your life doesn't mean you have to make sweeping changes. Whether it's realizing that every meal doesn't need to be home-cooked, or that you don't need to maintain the same weight as you did in high school, this transitional period is a time to cut yourself some slack.

This may also be a good point in your life to take some "me" time. If you've always wanted to take a yoga class, you'll find that it can reduce stress as well as strengthen your body. Perhaps you've wanted to reduce the hours you spend at work every day. Use your wisdom and mind power to envision a plan, and then make it work! Many people talk and write about the power of the feminine mind, but we don't even need to explore that here. Simply take some time for yourself and consider your short- and long-term goals and dreams. If you're like most women, your own needs have been put on the back burner for a while. Revisit them. Write them down. Make them happen.

Ask Yourself . . .				
Do you . . . with (fill in the blanks)	***Family***	***Relationships***	***Work***	***Yourself***
. . . have a problem saying no?	yes	yes	no	yes
. . . spend time?	yes	no	yes	no

Keep this in mind as you embark upon the program: everything in moderation. The goal of this program is to improve the condition of your health and well-being, not to create undue stress by adding another series of "to dos" to your list. That's why the word *balance* will continue to reappear throughout this book. By learning the tools to balance your life—and your hormones—you'll be better equipped to manage perimenopause.

Working with the Program

This specially designed program provides you with a guideline for making the perimenopausal transition with the fewest physical and emotional obstacles. But remember, it is merely a guideline and is not meant to take the place of advice and guidance by your physician or health care practitioner. In fact, this program was designed to complement your relationship with your health care provider. Take this book with you to your next office visit and discuss its topics with your doctor. If you don't have a doctor with whom you're comfortable, this is the time to look for a supportive, knowledgeable medical provider.

How to Choose a Doctor or Health Care Practitioner

An essential part of the program is finding a doctor or other health care professional who shares your values about health and healing. If you don't already have such a person in your life, now is the time to begin looking. A positive relationship built on trust between patient and practitioner can strongly influence the healing process. Conversely, negative, discouraging statements from a doctor may inhibit recovery.

Your chances of finding a suitable partner for your health care will greatly increase if you take charge of your own health and understand that you, alone, have the power to maintain your well-being. The role of the doctor/practitioner is to help provide you with the tools and knowledge necessary for *you* to do that effectively.

With the burgeoning popularity of health maintenance organizations (HMOs) and preferred provider organizations (PPOs), your job may be challenging. Some health care plans do not guarantee that you will see the same doctor from visit to visit. However, you can request a certain doctor and the chances are often good that your request will be honored. Remember that you don't always have to pay a lot of money to find a qualified, sympathetic doctor. If you ask the right questions thoughtfully and respectfully, more often than not this treatment will be reciprocated.

Often the best place to begin your search is by asking trusted friends or colleagues for a recommendation. The next step is to set up an appointment to talk to this person.

SEVERAL QUESTIONS TO ASK YOUR PROSPECTIVE DOCTOR

Remember that your doctor works for you and that *your* needs come first. After all, it's your body and you're paying the bill! Here are some good questions to ask your doctor:

- What are your beliefs surrounding perimenopause/menopause?
- Do you support a woman's need for preventive therapies?
- Can you help me regulate/adjust my diet, if necessary? If not, can you refer me to an appropriate person?
- Do you work with natural medicines? If not, do you support my decision to do so?
- Have you been trained in the use/efficacy of complementary therapies?
- Have you prescribed natural progesterone before? What have been the results?

- Can I call you if I have any questions? How difficult are you to reach?

If you are satisfied with the answers you receive, ask the most important question of all: Will you be my partner in my health care?

Journaling Your Way Back to Health

It would certainly make life easier if we could define perimenopause in a neat, clear-cut way. But we can't. Each woman reading this book is going to have a very different experience, and, in order to create the protocol that best meets *your* needs, you'll want to keep a journal.

As we begin to define the six-step protocol, you'll read about suggested treatments that you may not have even heard of before. This book will help you make the healthy transition—both mentally and physically—by educating you about the possibilities and offering you practical examples for using each step. We'll provide information about the mind/body connection. We'll talk about depression. We'll make suggestions for healthy eating that will promote well-being and fight the symptoms associated with perimenopause. We want you to understand how the different parts of your body work together to create the whole, and we'll support the fact that "fitness" is not just physical.

The program you design for your unique needs will, hopefully, encourage physical health, while also inviting more emotional, mental, and spiritual flexibility. If you want to improve the quality of your life, you will most likely have to make some lifestyle changes. You probably have already. That may include committing to an exercise program that feels great and works for you; letting go of self-judgment; changing your attitude about how, what, and when you eat; releasing anger; embracing your power; finding or recommitting to a spiritual path; and taking responsibility for how you feel physically and emotionally. Ultimately, it may mean recognizing that you are choosing the life you live.

We're not saying this program is going to be easy all of the time. As part of facing your mental challenge and preparing yourself for the tasks ahead, you might want to keep a journal. You don't have to let anyone else read it. This is for you only, so be fully open with yourself. It's a very important tool for keeping track of your attitude, progress, fears and doubts, feelings about certain activities, and more. Think of it as a best friend who is sitting before you, ears peeled, wanting to hear everything you go through. You can complain, you can rejoice, and you can go on endlessly about nothing. As you give yourself to your journal, you'll become more aware of what's going on within you while recording the progress you make outwardly.

Every person keeps a journal differently. Some women find it helpful to date each entry and update their journal daily, whereas others write in it more sporadically. There is no correct way to journal—the whole idea is to express yourself your way. However, for the purposes of this book, you'll want to keep track of certain things, such as what makes you feel better or worse and how you feel on certain days.

You may want to share what's inside the journal with friends and loved ones, or you may not. You decide. But you should write in it frequently and read it every now and then. Be sure it's compact enough to carry with you in case you'd rather read it in the privacy of a park or library. We advise against chalkboards as well as tiny notepads.

Setting Goals

At some point before you get into the rhythm of your program, you need to think about and write down your goals. If you've never been a goal-oriented person, don't let this scare you. Goals are simply landmarks of progress. They are the end of a certain journey and the beginning of another. They simply let you know that you are at a juncture. They're also good for measuring accomplishments. Write down several goals in your journal that you'd like to reach, for example:

1. I want to reverse my (fill in the blank) symptom.
2. I want to have more energy.
3. I want to meet other people who are committed to health and fitness so that I can be inspired.

Once you've recorded your goals, look at them and decide realistically when you think they can be achieved. Write how many weeks or months you think it will take and a "goal date" for having attained them, for example:

1. I want to reverse my symptoms (2 to 4 months).
2. I want to have more energy (1 year).
3. I want to meet other people who are committed to health and fitness so that I can be inspired (2 to 6 weeks).

After you've thoroughly explored these goals, go over them and decide which are the most important and which can be attained the soonest. Make two lists. Read them daily, especially before exercising.

The goals may change, and that's fine. But always have these two lists of goals close at hand: one with the most important goals no matter how long it will take to attain them and the other with goals that can be attained in the shortest amount of time. Once you've achieved one of the goals on your short-range list, replace it with another goal. As you cross the old ones off your list, reward yourself with something wonderful (flowers, a double feature, a weekend trip to a spa, a new bike—you get the picture).

Charting Your Symptoms

The second step in the program is to take inventory of your symptoms, when they occur, and how often they occur. You can use a blank page in your journal, or you can create a series of entries like the ones in the Basic Symptoms chart on page 41. Format is not important, but your attention to detail is essential.

If, after you've listed your symptoms, you want to write more, go ahead and do it. Remember that the purpose of the journal is to record physical changes and experiences, but also, and perhaps primarily, to provide a place in which you can vent, express, rant, cheer, explore—anything you want to do to keep the emotional, mental, and spiritual channels clear.

Introducing the Program

Once you've planned to balance your life and found a doctor who will be your partner in this program, you're ready to get started. The following basic components of your wellness plan will be outlined in detail in the subsequent chapters.

Step 1: Cleanse Your Liver

Lots of health programs say that you must first cleanse your liver. But what does that really mean and why is it so important?

The liver is the organ that works full-time to process the body's waste—and it gets no rest. Once you begin to experience the hormonal ups and downs of perimenopause , your liver may not be working at its optimum. Reducing stress to this vital organ is key at this time.

Chapter 4 will explain how the liver works and will provide you with a variety of tools for detoxifying it. You can choose a variety of easy techniques, from a basic liver tonic to improve liver function to a short-term fast for cleansing and energy enhancement.

Basic Symptoms							
List of Symptoms by Day and Time	*Monday*	*Tuesday*	*Wednesday*	*Thursday*	*Friday*	*Saturday*	*Sunday*
Irritability		3 P.M.		12 noon, 2 P.M.		11 A.M., 6 P.M., 7:30 P.M.	

Step 2: Consider Natural Progesterone

Many of the so-called problems that we associate with menopause—and that begin to surface during perimenopause—are caused by an imbalance of estrogen, progesterone, and testosterone. For example, the ovaries begin to decrease their production of estrogen, released during the menstrual cycle, and progesterone, released after ovulation. The decline of progesterone may occur first. Studies have shown that an increase in natural progesterone can balance the hormonal changes and, among other things, reduce the risk of osteoporosis.

Chapter 5 will explain how natural progesterone works. You'll also learn about the different types of progesterone, where to get them, and how best to use progesterone for your individual needs.

Step 3: Follow Dietary Recommendations

There are a variety of reasons to modify your diet during perimenopause, such as feeding your heightened nutritional needs and reducing the likelihood of various serious diseases, for example, heart disease, hypothyroidism, osteoporosis, and breast cancer.

Chapter 6 will discuss many foods that boost health and vitality and will offer suggestions for integrating these foods into your diet. Today, a back-to-basics approach to eating is considered the best way to address many health conditions. Additionally, foods with unique benefits will be explored as well as foods, cooking herbs, and spices that can help reduce or reverse perimenopausal symptoms. For example, iron-rich foods such as grains, nuts, seeds, and legumes assist liver function and offer efficient sources of energy. Soy products are an excellent replacement for meat and contain proteins that have been found to help in preventing osteoporosis. Foods containing phytohormones can help stabilize hormone fluctuations, thus reducing your symptoms.

Although this plan may sound intimidating, it's not. You don't need to throw out everything in your cupboards. Instead, you'll learn a variety of ways to integrate healthy foods into your diet and how to make healthier choices when shopping and dining out.

Step 4: Use Nutritional and Herbal Supplements to Balance Your Body and Reverse Symptoms

There are so many types of supplements on the market that, like most consumers, you're probably confused. Every day, it seems, a new supplement hits the market. Each one promises to be *the one* for your needs. What should you do?

It's certainly true that nutritional and herbal supplements can reverse perimenopausal symptoms and strengthen your body. Yet it's important to know how they work, what will work for you, and how to avoid taking the wrong supplement or too much or too little. Chapter 7 will explore the importance of regular supplementation, including how to choose a good multivitamin for your individual needs, and supplements for short-term and condition-specific needs, such as breast tenderness, hot flashes, and irregular menstrual periods.

Homeopathic remedies are another effective option in balancing perimenopausal symptoms. Although some remedies can be self-selected with little study, this is usually an area where professional consultation yields a better choice.

Meticulous journaling will really help you with this step. As you begin to supplement your program with nutritional and herbal medicine, chart the results carefully. Note if you feel better using a single supplement or with combinations. Do your symptoms subside or increase? Is your energy level better or worse?

Step 5: Exercise!

Any type of exercise you enjoy, whether it's yoga or long-distance running, releases endorphins from the endocrine system. Not only do these natural substances aid in balancing already delicate hormones, but endorphins also encourage a sense of mental and emotional well-being that can help reduce stress.

Weight-bearing exercise such as walking and movement therapies such as yoga or tai chi not only increase cardiovascular strength, they also have been shown to increase bone density and actually reverse the early signs of osteoporosis. Chapter 8 will discuss the various forms of exercise, their benefits, and how you can best integrate exercise and movement into your individual program.

Step 6: Expand Your Own Mind/Body Connection

Although women in perimenopause often menstruate, can generally conceive, and are not facing menopause for some time, the stigma attached to this term can stir up a host of emotional issues. These fears and concerns can be counterproductive to your health and well-being. Mind/body medicine teaches you how to use your mind as a healing tool to improve your overall health and reverse symptoms. Chapter 9 will help you identify the mind/body techniques you'll be most comfortable with and will provide instructions on how to use them.

CHAPTER FOUR

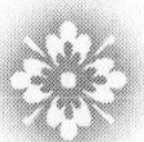

Cleanse Your Liver: Detoxification

The very first step to your program is the strange-sounding task of liver detoxification. Why is cleansing your liver so important? Even though we don't commonly talk about this, the liver is your primary organ for detoxification. Any substance that enters your body, whether it is through the mouth, skin, or nose, is filtered through the liver prior to its elimination.

As your body begins its hormonal roller coaster during perimenopause, your liver is additionally taxed by processing the higher levels of hormones excreted. A simple form of detoxification, dietary changes, or a formulated cleanse can reduce your symptoms and can assist your body in better processing the good materials you plan to put into it.

Note: No form of liver cleansing, no matter how simple it sounds, should be undertaken without first consulting with your doctor or practitioner. Not only is it important to assess your level of health prior to a detox, but harmful toxins can be released into the body during this cleansing, and you must have the medical support and knowledge to best deal with this process. Simple dietary changes, however, can be done independently and are a good way to see how you feel.

Why Detoxification?

Your body is a complex organism in constant interaction with a complex world. It is constantly repairing itself in a process of healthy homeostasis. It is designed to intake fuel, use the fuel to generate energy, and expel what it can't use through your liver, kidneys, urine, feces, exhalation, and perspiration. This is nature's method of detoxification.

Yet, as we have striven toward "progress," our industrial societies are giving off more waste than the earth can handle. Some of these toxic by-products are absorbed by our systems faster than we can eliminate them. The results, among others, are heightened estrogen levels during perimenopause, greater incidences of imbalances such as premenstrual syndrome, and larger reports of infertility.

Today, we are exposed to chemicals in far greater amounts than ever before. For example, over 69 million Americans live in areas that exceed smog standards; most drinking water contains more than 700 chemicals, including excessive levels of lead; some 3000 chemicals are added to the food supply; and as many as 10,000 chemicals in the form of solvents, emulsifiers, and preservatives are used in food processing and storage—all of which can remain in the body for years.

To compound these concerns, it isn't always possible to trace where your food comes from. While processed foods such as spaghetti sauce may seem clearly labeled, the label won't indicate where the tomatoes were grown, what types of pesticides were used in the fields, and if preservatives were added before packaging.

According to environmental medicine specialist William Ray, M.D., of Dallas, Texas, the buildup in the body of toxic substances, also called *bioaccumulation*, can seriously compromise your physiological and psychological well-being. Many of the symptoms experienced during perimenopause are exaggerated or worsened by this buildup, according to the hundreds of studies conducted on this subject.

About 20% of the population experiences negative effects from environmental pollutants. But you don't have to feel the negative effects for them to be present. Clinical studies have revealed that these toxins can be an extreme drain on your system, your body's stored nutrients in particular, regardless of whether you have noticeable symptoms.

The most common offenders are pesticides, which create a wide range of neurotoxicities in women. Other culprits are phenyls from plastics and formaldehyde from pressed boards, plywood, new carpets, and different synthetics. "Chlorine is a big offender, also," says Dr. Ray. "A lot of people report getting weak in their showers or after they drink chlorinated water."

These toxic chemicals tend to reside in the organs, particularly the reproductive organs, which is why a lot of women have severe premenstrual syndrome, have trouble conceiving or maintaining a pregnancy, and go into menopause early or have dramatic menopausal symptoms. These chemicals are also partly responsible for the heightened estrogen levels that occur during perimenopause.

As one option, many doctors suggest a home detox. You can start small, for example, by taking up the carpeting in the bedroom so that there are just hardwood floors. If possible, it's also advised to stay away from pressed wood or plywood in the bedroom and to sleep on an organic cotton futon or mattress.

Next, you may choose to look into carrying this cleansing throughout your entire living environment. Some experts advise you to try to stay away from gas heaters, using electric or hot water heat instead, and to use filtered air and drink filtered or distilled water in glass bottles, not plastic. These can be dramatic changes for some and you may or may not wish to explore these changes. There are many good resources in bookstores and on the Internet for helping you to create a healthier living/working environment.

Benefits of Detoxification

Choosing a method of detoxification that is right for you is part of the process. While special cleansing programs are key to rejuvenating the body and have been found to reduce the symptoms of perimenopause, it is important to have a full understanding and acceptance of how they work before agreeing to undergo any form of detoxification.

Because our diets today are taken from mineral-depleted, chemical-saturated farmlands and our meats are pumped up with excessive hormones, our bodies are armored with excess toxins that override many natural immune and detoxification abilities. By cleansing our bodies of these waste products, we can help restore well-being and optimal health.

There are many hormonal irregularities caused by toxic chemicals. They are manifested in such wide-ranging conditions as heart irregularities, asthma, brain dysfunction, headaches, bladder infections, and yeast infections. These health conditions, among others, are an indication that the body may need detoxification. Additionally, skin eruptions such as eczema, psoriasis, and acne can also indicate the need for a detox program.

Your doctor or practitioner may recommend laboratory tests to detect imbalances. These tests can analyze your stools, urine, blood, and hair to assess liver function and detect food allergies and are useful in many other health analyses. However, physicians who are not familiar with detoxification may be wary or reluctant to perform such tests. If you are considering a detoxification program, you will want to find a doctor or practitioner who understands and embraces this procedure. Great care must be taken to ensure the safe and effective removal of toxins, and detoxification therapy should be administered only after a consultation with a qualified health professional.

HEALING FROM THE INSIDE OUT

Detoxification is a good time for you to look inside and evaluate who you are, what is important to you, what you want to move toward, and what you want to let go of. Many women have found it helpful to start a journal or to begin some other type of creative process when going through detoxification. If journaling isn't for you, try listening to different types of music, exploring new areas of self-expression, or simply taking a long walk or a visit to a new place.

Whether the detox program finds you exhilarated or exhausted, it's a good time to harvest insights and inner wisdom. Pursue these outlets and understand that when your body is eliminating the toxins that have been clogging your mind, you will have better access into the psyche and you may learn some new things about your world.

Types of Detoxification

While each doctor or practitioner will have his or her own protocol for detoxification, this book will give you an overview of several methods most commonly practiced and how they can work individually or interactively.

Basic Dietary Changes

To get the most out of any detoxification program and to maintain benefits, you'll need to make some dietary changes. When a patient comes in with any type of system imbalance, a responsible doctor or practitioner will suggest making some basic nutritional adjustments. For many women this is really difficult because it can be time-consuming. Of course, these changes will take some time and effort, but diet is the quickest and easiest way to find some relief of your perimenopause symptoms and it provides you with a stronger foundation from which to fully detoxify your system. A more detailed explanation of a healing nutritional program will be outlined in Chapter 6.

Bowel Cleansing

After diet, the next easiest method of detoxification is evaluating the amount of fiber in your diet and increasing the amount to about 20 to 30 grams a day. For most people, fiber is a broom to their intestinal tract. It decreases the transit time of the toxins, eliminating them faster and actually cleaning the lining of the intestinal tract.

Until your bowels are moving and cleansing, your liver and other eliminatory organs will recycle these toxins back into the bowels, and they will be reabsorbed into more cells and tissues than they were originally. It's really amazing that a lot of physicians say to their patients, "It doesn't matter how often your bowels move. It's okay if they move once or twice a week." In a truly healthy body, on a high-fiber and healthy diet, bowels will move between one and three times a day. Every time they do, they are eliminating the toxins that would otherwise sit around and be reabsorbed. And since your reproductive organs are surrounded by bowels, they end up sharing the circulation and the recirculation of those toxins, which may very well increase the likelihood of health problems, including during perimenopause.

Fiber can come from many sources such as fruits, vegetables, and whole grains. Rice bran is a wonderful source of fiber. A cup of cooked beans usually has about 6 grams of fiber in it. Sometimes it's in cereals. If you need more fiber in your diet, it's easy to add some rice bran to your breakfast cereal. You can also sprinkle it on a salad, put it in soup, mash it in a potato, or mix it in a veggie burger.

Although oat bran is very popular, it shouldn't be used exclusively. It's a soluble fiber, and ideally you should use a mixture of soluble and insoluble fibers. Rice bran is ideal because it's a mixture of both. Another great way to increase fiber and essential fatty acids is to take psyllium seeds: grind them freshly and sprinkle them on foods without cooking them.

While increasing your fiber, remember to increase your water intake. Often, when you increase fiber, you may feel gassy and bloated for a couple of days. Understand that this change is temporary while your body is adjusting to the transition.

Liver Cleansing

There are many basic types of liver cleanses that can be done at home without constant medical supervision. Most of these are available over the counter at health food stores or natural pharmacies and are a combination of digestive enzymes and mild herbal laxatives. You should follow instructions carefully and cease use if you feel light-headed or more than very moderate abdominal discomfort.

Many practitioners use a liver-cleansing formula called Metabolic Formula that is filled with herbs for assisting the liver in cleaning itself out. Digestive enzymes help with the detoxification process and can be easily obtained at health food stores and many pharmacies.

High-intensity papaya and pineapple digestive enzymes can be beneficial if taken with meals. Two to four capsules are usually taken with each meal and can dramatically improve the body's cleansing process. If you are planning a detoxification fast (see below), these liver-cleansing aids should be taken for 1 to 3 months prior to the fast.

Fasting

According to Steven Bailey, N.D., of Portland, Oregon, "Fasting improves general liver function, which is not only removing toxins but converting and neutralizing them—the estrogen and progesterone hormones—specifically, the natural estrogen conversion that takes place in the liver." As a broad single-approach stimulant for your body working more efficiently, "very few things work as well as a good type of fasting program," he adds.

Although it may seem extreme to the uninitiated, a modified fast is a very natural method of detoxification. Instead of packing and jamming your blood full of toxins, you're cleaning out your blood and eliminating the waste products that have been backing up over months and years.

Dr. Bailey likens this process to a fire grate being full of ashes because the fire didn't completely burn the wood and ashes fell below the grate. When the grate gets clogged, the oxygen can't get in and keep the fire hot. This is similar to what happens in our cellular machinery. Those backed-up waste products smoulder away at our well-being, facilitating disease and accelerating aging by making the body work harder at its daily functions.

For perimenopausal women, Dr. Bailey usually recommends a 3- to 5-day juice fast. This length doesn't seem intimidating, so you're much more inclined to be successful if the fast is only a few days. A 2- to 3-day bulking period, in which you will consume a large variety of raw fruits and vegetables, precedes the fast. During the fast, 3 quarts of organic juice is consumed a day—2 quarts of vegetable juice (not carrot) and 1 quart of fruit juice mixed with water (a 50/50 mixture). At least 3 additional quarts of purified water ups the total to no less than 6 quarts of liquid consumed every day of the fast.

On the first day, you will probably struggle with the concept of not eating food, but you will also realize how full and satisfied you are. On the second day, your metabolism will be shifting and you may feel a bit cranky and fatigued. During the fast, Dr. Bailey encourages making time for a nap and not pushing yourself. You may not feel great as the toxins begin to pour out of your body. It's just the cleansing process. On the third day, you will probably feel better than you have in years and will not understand why you are not hungry, which might make it easier to go on to a fourth day and maybe a fifth.

IMPORTANT FASTING INFORMATION

Short weekend fasts, as described, are generally safe for most people, although you should seek advice from an appropriate health care professional experienced in detoxification—especially if you are considering your first fast. Longer fasts require medical supervision as well as prior assessment of levels of nutrients, such as vitamins and minerals, to ensure that deficiency does not occur.

Lymphatic Drainage

Lymphatic fluid circulates throughout the lymphatic system, carrying waste from all parts of the body. For women, the most obvious area of lymphatic blockage is the breasts. Castor packs applied directly to the breasts to facilitate drainage is suggested regardless of whether there is a problem. Castor oil packs can be made simply by soaking washcloths in castor oil. Squeeze out, then apply.

Jack Shields, M.D., a lymphologist from Santa Barbara, California, conducted a study on the effects of breathing on the lymphatic system. Using cameras inside the body, he found that deep diaphragmatic breathing stimulated the cleansing of the lymph system by creating a vacuum effect that sucked the lymphatic fluid through the bloodstream. This increased the rate of toxic elimination by as much as 15 times the normal pace. This type of breathing can be formally integrated into your lifestyle during yoga practices or a variety of other movement therapies (see Chapter 9).

Massage is also a powerful cleansing tool for lymphatic fluid, as is exercise. Water exercise, in particular, offers a good lymphatic massage. Swim or exercise in the water for 20 minutes and you'll get a natural lymphatic massage. Additionally, any vigorous aerobic exercise will accelerate lymphatic flow.

DETOXIFICATION SUPPORT

You can do a number of things while undergoing detoxification therapy to aid the natural cleansing ability of the body.

The boosts include:

Hydrotherapy: Epsom salts baths or wet sheet packs, once weekly.

Skin brushing: To assist the skin elimination function, daily.

Stretching and relaxation exercises: Daily.

Aerobic exercise (if appropriate): Brisk walking, jogging, dancing, etc., daily, except during the fast period.

Massage: Every other day during the detox, if possible.

Aromatherapy: Use appropriate (to your condition) aromatherapy oils in baths or as part of massage.

Breathing, relaxation, and meditation: Daily for at least 10 to 15 minutes, twice daily if possible.

CHAPTER FIVE

Consider Natural Progesterone

By now you understand the changes your body is going through and you've already learned the importance of detoxifying. Your next step is exploring natural progesterone and incorporating it into your program. This chapter will give you detailed guidelines. In addition, you'll learn why transdermal (through the skin) creams may be the best form for perimenopause, how to use them, and how to measure the results.

Many of the changes that begin to surface during perimenopause are caused by an imbalance of estrogen, progesterone, and testosterone. Symptoms can include water retention, loss of libido, weight gain, moodiness and irritability, and depression, as well as extreme manifestations such as breast cancer or endometrial cancer. Although estrogen production during perimenopause declines, the problems women experience are actually the results of too much estrogen. These problems, including fibrocystic breasts, breast tenderness and swelling, heavier or irregular periods, ovarian cysts, unexplained weight gain, and mood swings, can result from an excess of estrogen (released during the menstrual cycle) relative to progesterone, which is released after ovulation. Unfortunately, women can suffer from these symptoms for several years before they reach menopause, when menstruation ceases completely.

Yet there's no need to be unduly worried about this imbalance because a remarkable natural substance can reverse your symptoms. In fact, more and more doctors and practitioners today understand and appreciate the benefits of natural progesterone. Unlike many of the so-called "magic bullet" treatments out there, natural progesterone is easy to use, can be obtained without a prescription, has no known side effects, and has been proven overwhelmingly effective in clinical studies.

Studies have shown that supplementation of natural progesterone can balance the hormonal changes and, among other things, reduce the risk of developing osteoporosis. According to the pioneering physician John R. Lee, M.D., author of *What Your Doctor May Not Tell You About Premenopause*, natural progesterone is the best remedy for balancing hormones and may actually prevent further symptoms from occurring during this transition.

Why Natural Progesterone?

With the increasing number of baby boomers reaching midlife, it's no wonder that the products catering to women seem overwhelming. There are herbal formulas, designed to relax and rejuvenate; soy combos to boost energy and reverse some symptoms; and many other products that make a wide variety of claims.

Yet, in many cases, perimenopausal women may need only natural progesterone to relieve all of their symptoms. Progesterone is a precursor molecule that the body can use to produce estrogens and androgens. In simple language, natural progesterone provides the fuel necessary for your body to regulate itself. Since there is no smarter or more efficient engine than the human body, it makes good sense to provide your body with the tool it needs for optimal health and efficiency. Additionally, natural forms of progesterone are inexpensive to manufacture, and you may find that natural progesterone is considerably less expensive than the synthetic progestins that some physicians still prescribe.

Progesterone is produced by all mammals. Although often referred to as a sex hormone, it conveys no secondary sex characteristics and as such cannot be categorized as exclusively masculine or feminine. It does, however, affect many body parts and functions, including the uterus, vagina, and cervix, the brain, metabolism, thyroid function, nerve function, energy production, the immune system, and fetal survival and growth. No wonder an imbalance can cause such wide-ranging chaos in your body!

According to William Ray, M.D., of Dallas, Texas, natural progesterone cream can offer relief from a variety of perimenopause symptoms. He tells the story of a woman who, all of a sudden, began feeling fatigued, weak, and depressed, and was experiencing memory loss. "We found out she had a hormone deficiency and she also started having premenstrual tension that she never had in her life. We prescribed a little progesterone. She found that every third day she seemed to need a little bit more. So she listened to her body and, on those days, applied about one third more of the cream, and returned to her primary dose for days one and two. And she's done very well."

Here's an added benefit: All women are concerned about the cumulative effects of osteoporosis (the thinning of bones, which can lead to fractures), which can begin to take its toll during the early 20s. This risk continues during perimenopause and beyond. In fact, after menopause, women tend to lose 2% to 4% of bone mass each year for about 10 years until the loss begins to level off, but by then much of the damage has already been done. Preliminary studies have reported that natural progesterone may be beneficial in stopping the effects of osteoporosis.

Why Natural Progesterone is Beneficial

Of all hormones, natural progesterone is the most important for your optimal health because:

- Natural progesterone helps use fat for energy.
- Natural progesterone is a natural antidepressant.
- Natural progesterone promotes restful sleep.
- Natural progesterone facilitates thyroid hormone activity.
- Natural progesterone normalizes blood sugar levels.
- Natural progesterone helps restore proper cell oxygen levels.
- Natural progesterone alleviates hormone-related migraine headaches.
- Natural progesterone is a natural diuretic (prevents water retention).
- Natural progesterone normalizes blood clotting.
- Natural progesterone normalizes monthly cycles.
- Natural progesterone helps protect against breast fibrocysts.
- Natural progesterone helps prevent breast cancer.
- Natural progesterone helps prevent endometrial cancer.
- Natural progesterone helps maintain the lining of the uterus.
- Natural progesterone stimulates osteoblast function (bone cell rebuilding).

- Natural progesterone helps protect against heart disease.
- Natural progesterone helps protect against environmental toxins.
- Natural progesterone helps restore normal libido.

June, who is 41 years old, began using natural progesterone cream after she was diagnosed with endometriosis. Her doctor initially suggested that she have a hysterectomy. When she insisted on exploring other alternatives, June was referred to another doctor, who prescribed natural progesterone. After 4 months of application, June's biopsy showed that her condition had reversed itself and all signs of the endometriosis had disappeared. At that time, June's doctor reduced her dose to a maintenance level, on which she currently remains.

Is Natural Progesterone Cream Therapy Safe?

If you haven't already heard of natural progesterone, you'll undoubtedly want to know the cons as well as the pros. Adverse side effects are rare and usually subside quickly with the reduction or cessation of use.

You may wonder why your doctor hasn't prescribed natural progesterone. Maybe you just need to ask. Many traditional medical doctors are in the process of discovering the many benefits of natural progesterone cream and its lack of side effects. Yet some are reluctant to prescribe it wholeheartedly. While approximately 40,000 medical doctors in the United States practice some form of complementary medicine, there are still many who are wary if the treatment is not a patented pharmaceutical product, in spite of the fact that it may be safe and effective. If this is the case with your doctor or practitioner, it may be your job to gently educate him or her.

When it comes to safety, synthetic forms of progesterone, called progestins, are another matter entirely. In fact, The *Physician's Desk Reference* details a long list of warnings, side effects, contraindications, and potential increased cancer risk associated with the use of all synthetic hormones. Disturbingly high levels of progestins are found in certain birth-control products. If you are using birth-control pills, creams, or gels, talk to your health care provider about their progestin levels.

What about Estrogen?

Perimenopausal women often ask if they need supplemental estrogen. It's most likely that your symptoms are caused by *estrogen dominance*, so there's really no need to add even more estrogen. Most women respond well to natural progesterone cream, especially when it is used with some important dietary modifications and lifestyle changes.

The use of a properly formulated progesterone cream is approximately half of a well-rounded approach to optimally balancing your hormones. The other half requires avoiding the chemicals that suppress the production and/or utilization of natural progesterone and are usually the underlying cause of hormone-related health problems. Most commercially grown meat and dairy contain synthetic hormones that are added by the grower for profit, as well as pesticide residues with some estrogenic properties. These chemical compounds are powerful in their activity and are largely responsible for low progesterone levels in women. We'll discuss this topic in more detail in Chapter 6.

Since progesterone is the biological precursor for estrogen, many women have found that they can achieve a normal balance between estrogen and progesterone by the use of a correctly formulated natural progesterone cream and the implementation of well-established dietary/lifestyle modifications.

The Side Effects of Estrogen Dominance

- Increased body fat
- Metabolism dysfunction
- Depression and headaches
- Salt and water retention
- Increased food cravings
- Reduced oxygen in all cells
- Decreased sex drive
- Excessive blood clotting
- Increased risk of breast cancer
- Increased risk of endometrial cancer
- Endometriosis
- Uterine cramping
- Infertility

The Best Form

Most American women take natural progesterone transdermally (applied to the skin), in the form of an over-the-counter cream, or orally, in the form of an oil. Many doctors and practitioners recommend the transdermal method over other options because of the efficient manner in which the body utilizes it. Here's the simplified version of what happens: as you rub the cream into your body, the progesterone is absorbed through the skin and is stored in your fat cells. As needed, the fat cells gradually release the progesterone and transmit it through your body's circulatory system to the progesterone receptor sites on your cells. Not only is the cream easy to use, but it is an effective way to manage symptoms for most women.

When estrogen and progesterone are released into the bloodstream by the ovaries, each is wrapped in a protein sheath. Estrogen is bound to sex hormone–binding globulin (SHBG) and progesterone is bound to cortisol-binding globulin (CBG). Fat-soluble, nonprotein-bound hormones do not mix well with the watery blood serum or plasma, so they are transmitted through the blood by attaching themselves to red blood cell membranes. When protein bound, they are water soluble. Only 2% to 10% of the progesterone in blood plasma is unbound and readily available for use. Less than 10% of the protein-bound hormone is active.

Transdermal progesterone works on your symptoms by passing through the skin and into the layer of fat that lies beneath the skin, known as subcutaneous fat. The more your body needs it, the more efficiently it will process the progesterone. Although transdermal progesterone given to a progesterone-deficient woman shows up right away in a saliva hormone test, it can take as long as 3 months for an increase to show up in blood tests. This gradual release achieved by transdermal progesterone is the only dosing method that approximates the natural physiologic release of the hormone from the ovaries.

Relief of symptoms is the most convincing proof that transdermal progesterone is indeed absorbed and distributed throughout the body. Extreme symptoms such as fibrocystic breasts have been reversed in merely 3 to 4 months after using progesterone cream transdermally. A recent study supports this clinical finding. In the study, over 1000 women used various combinations of hormone creams before surgery to remove breast cysts. The results showed that breast tissue levels of progesterone increased 100 times, and estrogen-induced stimulation of breast cell proliferation (the first step toward breast cancer growth) was significantly inhibited after just 8 to 10 days of using transdermal progesterone.

Uses for Oral Progesterone

While we recommend the transdermal form of progesterone for the treatment of perimenopausal symptoms, another common form is oral. When natural progesterone is administered orally in a capsule, it is in the form of micronized progesterone. Although oral progesterone may be less effective in treating the perimenopausal symptoms in some women, it can be quite effective for others. However, this is an issue best determined after careful examination of your symptoms by your physician. Oral progesterone has also been found to be effective in the treatment of hormone-related migraine headaches. If this is one of your symptoms, you should discuss this with your doctor or health care practitioner.

How to Select a Progesterone Cream

Only a few of the progesterone creams on the market actually have proven levels of progesterone. For example, despite many statements to the contrary, the popular supplement wild yam cannot deliver progesterone through the skin. Pioneering physician John Lee, M.D., author of the best-selling *What Your Doctor May Not Tell You about Premenopause* and *What Your Doctor May Not Tell You about Menopause*, states "There is no evidence that the human body converts diosgenin (found in Mexican wild yam) to hormones."

It's important to know that all natural progesterone is not created equal. Progesterone products that contain the semi-synthetic hormone are much more potent—up to 30 times—than those containing progesterone precursors from plants. To put this in perspective, synthetic progestins are about 10 to

100 times as potent as the progesterone made by your body! Some of the precursors in these products have estrogenic qualities as well. The stronger natural progesterone preparations, such as micronized progesterone pills, tend to be available only by prescription. The exact amounts of the hormones in some brands of natural progesterone are considered to be proprietary. However, a recent Food and Drug Administration (FDA) regulation requires that companies put the word *progesterone* on the label if the compound includes the active hormone, so you can check to see if a product is more or less potent.

For effectiveness, a transdermal cream should contain no less than 400 mg progesterone per ounce. The following creams meet or surpass this standard: ProGest, Fem-Gest, Bio Balance, Ostaderm, Progonol, ProBalance, and Serenity. All the dosage recommendations in this chapter are based on using a 2-ounce container of progesterone cream that contains a total of 960 mg of progesterone. This amounts to 40 mg per ½ teaspoon, 20 mg per ¼ teaspoon, and 10 mg per ⅛ teaspoon. There is virtually no danger of overdose, and many women use the equivalent of an entire tube or jar per week with no ill effects. There are creams available that offer extreme doses of progesterone (3000 mg or more per 2-ounce jar), which you should avoid because the content is too high to effectively manage.

HORMONE LEVEL TESTING

As we'll discuss later, the best way to gauge your success with natural progesterone cream is by the relief and/or reversal of symptoms. However, this type of thinking doesn't mesh well with the ways conventional doctors generally monitor results.

Many doctors believe that progesterone creams don't work because they don't result in high blood levels. Protein-bound progesterone is more soluble in the watery component of the blood. While protein bound, only a small percentage of the hormone is active. This is also true of estrogens, testosterone, and the corticosteroids. For this reason, blood serum concentration of these hormones is not an accurate measure of the amount of active hormone in the body because it misses the larger amount that is riding on red blood cell membranes.

Serum levels of progesterone are often low when a woman is on progesterone creams because when progesterone is absorbed into the bloodstream, 80% of it will be bound to the plasma membranes of the red blood cells—the part that is thrown out when serum levels are checked. This is also why salivary levels of hormones often measure higher than serum levels. Ideally, your doctor or practitioner will be aware of this fact and, if he or she is intent on monitoring your hormone levels for results, will choose saliva testing over blood.

The good news is that transdermal progesterone maintains stable saliva levels for 8 hours or more after application. Thus, if you're applying 15 to 20 mg of progesterone cream daily, your saliva levels should maintain a constant level throughout a 24-hour period.

The Right Stuff: It's All a Matter of Dose

Now that you understand how natural progesterone works, you're probably eager to incorporate it into your program. How much should be taken and how often it should be used are probably the most common questions addressed to doctors. Every woman is unique. In fact, in just about every aspect of their physiology, women differ. Not only do we not all look and behave the same, our metabolism and physiology can greatly differ. It's bad medicine to give a blanket dose to everyone, regardless of medication, and natural progesterone is no exception.

Although your doctor or practitioner will give you an approximate dosage to begin with, based on your medical evaluation, ultimately you must find the best amount for your body. The dosage for creams varies according to the type of cream you use, the severity of the symptoms, and the reason you're using it. Therefore, it's important to consult with a doctor or practitioner *before* using the natural progesterone cream. The chart on page 69 will help you and your health care practitioner track how your symptoms respond to the cream.

Your goal will be to find and use the minimum amount you need to obtain relief from your symptoms. You may need to use a bit more at first (especially if your symptoms are severe), but you'll want to experiment with dosages as you become accustomed to using the cream. The good news is that you can't do anything wrong. Natural progesterone is so safe that you won't experience serious side effects if you end up using a bit more than your body needs. This gives you a window to find your best dose.

The Initial Dose

For the first 3 or 4 months, you should use the natural progesterone cream for 12 to 18 days, with 3 to 4 days off between these cycles. Based on your doctor's evaluation, you will most likely be given an initial dose of between 10 and 40 mg per day.

Since the more common brands come in 2-ounce jars containing 960 mg of progesterone, here's an easy breakdown: 40 mg per ½ teaspoon, 20 mg per ¼ teaspoon, and 10 mg per ⅛ teaspoon. If your measurements are off by a little, don't worry; the goal will be to use one third to one half the container per month, until your symptoms reverse or you and your doctor decide to modify the protocol.

Using Natural Progesterone Cream

List of Treatment by Day and Time	*Monday*	*Tuesday*	*Wednesday*	*Thursday*	*Friday*	*Saturday*	*Sunday*
Week 1	1/8 tsp. No change	1/8 tsp. No change	1/8 tsp. No change	1/8 tsp. No change	1/8 tsp. No change	1/8 tsp. No change	1/4 tsp. No change
Week 2	1/4 tsp. No change	1/4 tsp. No change	1/4 tsp. No change	1/4 tsp. No change	1/4 tsp. Better	1/4 tsp. Better	1/4 tsp. Better
Week 3	1/4 tsp. Better	1/4 tsp. Better	1/4 tsp. Better	1/4 tsp. Better	1/4 tsp. Better	1/4 tsp. Better	1/4 tsp. Good
Week 4							
Week 5							
Week 6							
Week 7							

Maintenance Dose

Over the course of about 3 to 4 months, the average woman with a progesterone deficiency will find that her symptoms will reverse. If your symptoms subside, you may want to reduce your dose by about 20% to see if you can maintain your hormonal balance. Whatever reverses your symptoms and restores a sense of well-being is the ideal dose for you.

The goal is not to stockpile progesterone but to achieve a balance in your hormones. Although your body may not react negatively in the form of side effects by taking a supercharged dose, the excess will be funneled out through your liver—unduly taxing the liver you just cleaned out! If you and your doctor determine the amount of progesterone that your body would normally produce and supplement accordingly and your symptoms still don't go away, it's best to return to your doctor or health care practitioner to figure out why.

Where and When to Apply

Where and when you decide to administer the progesterone cream is up to you, but most doctors recommend using the cream first thing in the morning and right before you go to bed at night. If you can't determine your exact dose, don't be too concerned. A slight bit too much or too little is not something to worry about—your body will regulate that extra bit. The key to restoring balance is in the regulated fueling of your system by the progesterone. Thus, missing a dose completely would be a greater deficit to your body.

For the best results when using a transdermal cream, apply it to the areas of your body with the thinnest skin: your chest, neck, face, and inner thighs. Try to spread it on a larger area of skin so that the cream can benefit from greater absorption by the skin. You should allow sufficient time for the cream to be absorbed, which is why bedtime is ideal. Do not apply the cream over another product, such as moisturizer, and do not use anything over the cream either. You should try to rotate the areas to which you apply the cream because continuous usage in one area will discourage proper absorption over time.

There are many quality natural progesterone creams available. If you can't find a pharmacy in your area that carries them, see the Where to Find Help section of this book.

CHAPTER SIX

Follow Dietary Recommendations

Although the word *diet* is no stranger to most women, it's surprising how few really know what good nutrition is. Many women have spent their adult lives on some sort of diet, concerning themselves with the way they look rather than the way they feel. For many it's a health crisis, such as that first hot flash or memory lapse, that jump starts them on the path to better eating. Good health, vitality, and even beauty come from a lifestyle that emphasizes good nutrition.

Whole foods not only fuel our bodies more efficiently but actually act as a tonic to balance the system. This healthful, balanced way of eating can improve health and even reverse symptoms of illness, just as poor eating habits can deteriorate the body and the mind.

In the United States and many other places in the world, the relationship between food and health is profoundly dysfunctional. The connection between what we eat and how we feel, although understood by many in principle, is lost upon most of us in practice. For women who have eaten erratically over the years, the whole-foods diet described in this chapter may seem like a dramatic change. Yet you'll be surprised how easy it is if you make the transition slowly. Whole foods simply taste better, fill you up more completely, and, over time, give you a higher level of energy and a greater sense of well-being. If you're already eating healthfully, you'll learn some tools in this chapter for modifying your diet to ease or reverse your perimenopause symptoms.

Keep a Journal

You're probably not aware of what you eat and how much. Now is your opportunity to become aware, at least for a few months.

Keep two journals if you prefer (one for food, the other for the purposes we discuss in other chapters). Record everything you eat and drink throughout the day. It may be easier to keep your food journal within sight of where you eat so that you don't forget to record what you put in your mouth. Don't worry about fat content or calories (unless, of course, you want to). Just write down:

1. What time it is
2. What you ate
3. How much you ate (i.e., small portion, medium portion, and so on)
4. How many you ate (one apple, three servings of mashed potatoes, and so on)
5. How you felt when you were eating
6. How you felt after you ate

The food journal could be used as a tool to judge and beat up the eater, which would be completely counterproductive; or it could be used to make you aware of how emotions play into eating habits and how your eating habits may be so ingrained that you aren't even aware of them. Use it to become aware. Use it so that you can know what you eat. Use it to help you reach your goals.

TREAT YOUR SYMPTOMS AND ALSO ENJOY . . .

A stronger immune system

When you start eating foods that nourish and strengthen your body, you'll not only feel better physically, you'll also have an improved outlook on life. In turn, your immune system will become stronger and better able to address the challenges caused during perimenopause. A strong immune system should be one of your top goals, and eating right, exercising, and being aware of the powerful mind/body connection will help bring you closer and closer to that goal.

A lowering of high blood pressure

Obesity and diets heavy in salt, alcohol, and fatty or sugary foods can bring on or aggravate high blood pressure and cholesterol levels. Those types of foods also increase the risk of stroke and heart disease. Although you may not be concerned about these conditions today, remember that heart disease is the number one disease risk of menopausal women. So get a jump on the competition and get healthy today.

Once you change your eating habits, monitor your cholesterol and blood pressure regularly, then enjoy the feeling of triumph when they start to drop!

Food Journal

List of Foods by Day and Time	*Monday*	*Tuesday*	*Wednesday*	*Thursday*	*Friday*	*Saturday*	*Sunday*

Take a Quick Inventory

If you're like the majority of women experiencing perimenopausal symptoms, it's probably because your diet is causing (or exacerbating) hormonal imbalances. Before you read through and attempt to tackle a new way of eating, take an inventory of your diet and eating habits.

Take out your journal and jot down what you've eaten, how much, and what you felt like during the meals. Do this daily for a week. How have you prepared the foods you've eaten? Do you bake, broil, or poach the foods, or sizzle them in oil? How about your portions—What determines the size? How much do you *want* to serve yourself? After reading your journal, do you find any patterns in how you feel in relation to what you eat?

Once you've done that, address some of your emotional issues surrounding food (and don't say they're not there—we all have them). Answer the following questions in complete sentences (no single-word answers, please!), and, most importantly, be honest with yourself:

1. Do you eat when you're emotional? If so, what are the dominant emotions that drive you to eat (pain, anger, depression, resentment, elation, jealousy, powerlessness, excitement)?
2. What are the foods that you crave when you're emotional?
3. Do you find comfort in those foods, or do they actually make you feel worse after you've eaten them?
4. Do you often eat when you're not hungry? How many times in your journal did you mention that you weren't hungry when you ate?
5. Could you call yourself addicted to a specific food or foods?

6. What is it about food that makes you want it? Does it fill up an emptiness inside you? Is it the taste that satisfies you? Does it remind you of something from the past that makes you feel good?
7. If you could direct your eating habits, when would you eat? How much? What kinds of foods?
8. Are you willing to give up eating certain foods (most of the time) that you love? If so, why? If not, why not?
9. Do you like to cook? If so, what do you like about it? If not, what do you dislike about it?

After you answer these questions, you'll undoubtedly be one step closer to gleaning new insights about your relationship to food. Keep writing and see where it takes you. If you feel that you could greatly benefit from digging a little deeper to discover what purpose food fulfills in your life (beyond providing fuel), do so. This step is important because your relationship with food may have a powerful hold over you and simply telling yourself to change your habits may not be enough to carry out a lasting change. You might need to heal a past pain, face a current one, or give up an insatiable need for instant gratification that's rooted in something you may not even understand.

Overeating, binge eating, or simply eating all the time is often a way for people to avoid their problems. Maybe you are on bad terms with your spouse or children. Maybe you're depressed about this life transition. Maybe you're not happy with yourself or your life situation. Or maybe your car didn't start this morning. Problems can be big or little, but turning to food is a typical "answer" for many people.

Be honest with yourself. If you aren't, the program will not work. If you suspect that food may be a problem for you, consider seeking professional help. There are counselors and therapists who specialize in eating disorders either in a group or individual setting and are discreet about treatment.

Part I What's Wrong with Our Diets

The typical American diet of the past few decades has been comprised of more processed and contaminated foods than ever before. At the same time, American women are increasingly suffering from more degenerative and autoimmune diseases, with studies proving an obvious link between poor eating habits and illness. Unfortunately, perimenopause is often a time when these dietary shortcomings are revealed. Because hormonal imbalances make your body more vulnerable and susceptible to the wide range of perimenopausal symptoms, a poor diet will only exaggerate this fact, whereas a healthful diet will reduce (and can even reverse) these discomforts.

Over the years, medical research has shown that saturated fats, white flour, refined starches, red meat, and chemical additives and pesticides—all common elements of the American diet—are major contributors to poor health and disease. "What we eat may affect our risk for several of the leading causes of death for Americans," stated the 1988 *Surgeon General's Report on Nutrition and Health*, "notably, the degenerative diseases such as atherosclerosis, coronary heart disease, strokes, diabetes, and some types of cancers. These disorders, combined, account for more than two-thirds of all deaths today in the United States."

Over the past decade, however, many of the myths that reinforced our eating habits have been exposed by the burgeoning health care (and health food) industry. Nevertheless, most of us cling to a diet that provides only a fraction of the nutrition our bodies require to function properly. Why do we continue to consume unhealthy food even in the face of potential illness? Many experts conclude that a strong emotional undercurrent must be driving our dietary choices. Nutritionist D. Lindsey Berkson, M.A., D.C., of Santa Fe, New Mexico, believes that lack of emotional well-being is perhaps the single greatest barrier to good nutrition, particularly for women.

Overcoming the emotional block that stands between good eating and good health can be a huge challenge. Many people are intimidated at the prospect of changing their eating habits, feeling that they must sacrifice pleasure or routine for some vague promise of better health. For many women, years of crash or elimination dieting has altered their perceptions of what is healthy: in their distorted view, only thin = healthy.

Many of these women deprive their bodies of good nutrition and suffer through premenstrual syndrome (PMS) symptoms for years until they transition into perimenopausal symptoms. Often, these women continue to suffer through hot flashes, depression, and memory fogs even though these symptoms could be managed through diet. It doesn't have to be an all-or-nothing approach. The goal is to strike a balance so that 75% to 80% of the time you are eating well, then allowing yourself some indulgences. Ultimately, good nutrition depends upon a holistic view of food—one that embraces the connection between physical, mental, and emotional health. For those who honor this relationship, the rewards can be great.

Repetition versus Variety in the Diet

Today's typical American diet contains too few foods. Unfortunately, most Americans eat the same foods meal after meal, only disguised by different names. They also consume food not according to what is best for them but according to what tastes best to them.

If you look closely, the American menu is actually made up of various combinations of the same foods, usually wheat, beef, eggs, potatoes, and milk products. For example, a breakfast of eggs, sausage, white toast, and hash browns is the same as a lunch of a hamburger, white bun, and fries, which is the same as a dinner of steak and potatoes or white pasta. Besides the fact that they are high-fat, high-calorie, low-fiber, and toxin-filled meals, they are strikingly devoid of fruits and vegetables. They are also low in many of the essential nutrients.

Daily consumption of the same foods tends to produce allergies and hypersensitivities to those foods, according to experts in environmental medicine. Instead of nourishing the body, these foods may start to act against it. Eating a varied diet minimizes these problems. The optimal diet should consist of more vegetables, fruits, and whole grains than any other foods.

The Whole-Foods Diet

Today, there's a wide consensus that Americans should consume far less fat, animal protein, and processed foods and eat more complex carbohydrates, especially whole grains rich in fiber, and at least five servings daily of fruits and vegetables. Buck Levin, Ph.D., R.D., assistant professor of nutrition at Bastyr College in Seattle, Washington, offers a simple prescription for a healthy diet: one of natural, whole foods. "By whole foods we mean consuming a diet that is high in foods as whole as possible, with the least amount of processed, adulterated, fried, or sweetened additives," says Dr. Levin.

A whole-foods diet is generously filled with a wide variety of different-colored vegetables, fruits, and grains; raw seeds and nuts and their butters; beans; fermented milk products such as yogurt and kefir; and fish, poultry, and soy products such as tofu. This diet is lower in animal meats, fats, and cheeses.

A sense of balance is important in approaching your diet. If the majority of meals are comprised of whole, fresh foods, then a little junk food, an occasional glass of wine, and a piece of cake here or there won't hurt. But when too few whole foods are consumed, the body's physiology is compromised.

The very concept of whole foods is foreign to many people. Products such as whole-wheat flour are often thought to be some health fanatic's variation on the real deal. Few understand that it is the other way around—that white bread, white rice, and other such foods are perversions of the original thing. A whole grain is exactly that—the bran, the germ, and the inside starch.

When you remove the bran, not only are you throwing away the fibers, you are also throwing away the B vitamins that are not really made up in other parts of your diet. You're also throwing away the germ with essential oils such as vitamins E and K. So when you eat the whole food, when you eat the whole grain, you don't have to think: What did I miss? It's already there as nature intended it. For example, when you have white rice, you miss the magnesium in the brown rice, and magnesium is critical for strengthening bones and preventing osteoporosis.

Freshness is another component of the whole-foods diet—buying produce straight from the farm and minimizing the consumption of frozen foods and preservatives. This may not be possible for most people, but the basic idea is sound. If possible, buy fresh. Choose fresh vegetables over frozen or canned and cook them in a way that preserves the most nutrients, such as steaming or stir-frying.

Although changing to a whole-foods diet might seem complicated, in fact it's just the reverse. You're eating foods that an ancestor would have recognized as food 200 years ago. The idea is that you're eating foods that haven't been processed, or they've been processed in such a minimal way that nutrients haven't been taken away that could be used in your body. And you're using foods that are fresh and have not been treated in any way that would put more chemicals into your body. You have a greater chance of remaining healthy.

Stressor Foods

A whole foods diet is low in stressor foods—those foods that rob the body rather than nourish it. Examples of stressor foods are refined sugars, commercial cola, refined grain flours and pastas, processed fats, hydrogenated fats such as margarine, and deep-fried foods. These foods can disturb the physiology of the body. For example, hydrogenated fats contain trans-fatty acids that inhibit normal essential fatty acid metabolism and may negatively affect liver function and blood fat levels. Refined sugars, when consumed in excess, decrease immune functioning, increase risk of heart disease and obesity, promote dental decay, aggravate hyperactive behavior in some children, and provide no nutritional value at all. Commercial colas are high in phosphates that deplete the body of calcium and, when consumed daily, put women at risk of osteoporosis (excessive loss of calcium from bones, causing spontaneous fractures and a marblelike appearance).

Margarine is a classic example of a stressor food. The process of turning normally liquid vegetable fat into a solid creates a trans-fatty acid—a substance that the human body never encountered prior to the invention of margarine. The substance is close enough to a regular fat that your membranes will absorb it and try to utilize it. It's a lot like putting motor oil in your gasoline tank: your car will recognize it as a liquid and circulate it through the engine, yet it lacks the capacity to generate energy. In short, you are better off eating small amounts of butter and limiting your total fat than using margarine, shortening, and other substitutes.

Processed foods often act as stressors because of the presence of chemical additives. In an effort to produce low-fat snack foods, we've created nutritionless products with more chemicals—and the chemicals are more of a problem than the fat would have been. In general, stay away from packaged foods, which are usually high in preservatives. If a food is preserved, make sure it's in its own juice or water and there is nothing added to it. If you'd like to learn more about the latest food products on the market, read *Nutrition Action*, a newsletter put out by the Center for Science in the Public Interest (see the section on Where to Find Help).

The Whole Oil Story

Much of the information on fats is confusing and even contradictory, so here's the whole story. There are three types of fats, or lipids, which are differentiated by their chemical makeup: saturated, monounsaturated, and polyunsaturated. The human body needs a certain amount of each of these lipids to function properly. Common fats and oils have components of all of them. For example, canola oil is 62% monounsaturated fat, 32% polyunsaturated fat, and 6% saturated fat.

Saturated Fats

Saturated fats are found primarily in animal foods and tropical oils such as coconut and palm oil. Due to their chemical structure, saturated fats tend to remain solid at room temperature. Although there is a tremendous amount of evidence that supports the relationship between high fat intake from animal sources and heart disease, some amount of saturated fat in the diet is necessary. Saturated fat is needed for the liver's production of cholesterol, an important component in the structure of cell membranes. In addition, stearic acid, one of the most common saturated animal fats, has been shown in some studies to be beneficial in fighting cardiovascular disease.

Monounsaturated Fats

Monounsaturated fats are considered healthier than polyunsaturated fats because of their ability to lower LDL (low-density lipoprotein, commonly called bad) cholesterol while maintaining or raising HDL (high-density lipoprotein, or good) cholesterol. Canola oil and olive oil are naturally high in monounsaturated fats.

Although the evidence is not ironclad, a study published in the *Journal of the American Medical Association* surveyed 4900 Italian men and women, whose ages ranged from 20 to 59, and found that those who had a diet high in olive oil and low in butter and margarine also had lower overall levels of cholesterol and blood pressure than those whose diets included more butter and margarine.

Polyunsaturated Fats

Plentiful in safflower, sunflower, and corn oil, polyunsaturated fats contain both omega-6 and omega-3 essential fatty acids (EFAs). Omega-6 is beneficial when a person is injured, causing blood to clot and blood vessels to constrict. In contrast, omega-3 inhibits harmful clotting, relaxes vascular smooth muscle, and has an antiarrhythmic effect, reducing the risk of heart disease.

Humans evolved on a diet that contained small but roughly equal amounts of omega-6 and omega-3 fatty acids. Then, about a century ago, the food supply began to change. The vegetable oil industry began to hydrogenate oil, which reduced the oil's omega-3 content. At the same time, the domestic livestock industry began to use feed grains, which happen to be rich in omega-6 fatty acid and low in omega-3. As a result, the American diet now has an EFA ratio of 20–25:1 omega-6 to omega-3, rather than the 1:1 ratio with which humans evolved. The modern diet is too high in omega-6, which may contribute to heart disease.

There are many foods that can boost the intake of omega-3 essential fatty acids. Fish is a good source, as well as beans, especially great northern, kidney, navy, and soy beans. In oils, omega-3 is most abundant in flaxseed, but there is also canola oil with a 10% omega-3 content and soy, pumpkin seed, evening primrose, borage seed, walnut, and black currant oils.

Part II Benefits of a Whole-Foods Diet

A whole-foods diet promotes health by decreasing fat and sugar intake and increasing fiber and nutrient intake. Ideally, it means more satisfaction and less overeating. The guidelines given later in this chapter for reversing your perimenopausal symptoms are based on a basic whole-foods eating plan. The following guidelines will help you achieve hormonal and nutritional balance through diet. Try different food combinations and see what works for you.

Eat More Fiber

Animal products, such as meat, cheese, milk, eggs, and butter contain no fiber, compared to brown rice, broccoli, oatmeal, and almonds, which have from 6 to 15 grams per serving. Fiber is the transport mechanism of the digestive tract, moving food wastes out of the body before they have a chance to form potentially cancer-causing chemicals. These toxic chemicals can cause colon cancer or pass through the gastrointestinal membrane into the bloodstream and damage other cells. You don't need to eat more food or consume more calories in order to eat more fiber, nor do you have to eliminate foods you like because they have less. Simply be aware of the fiber content of foods you eat and make better choices overall or consider a fiber supplement such as wheat bran or psyllium seed husks .

Consume Less Fat

On a percentage-of-calories basis, most vegetables contain less than 10% fat, and most grains contain from 16% to 20% fat. By comparison, whole milk and cheese contain 74% fat. A rib roast is 75% fat, and eggs are 64% fat. Low-fat milk or a skinned, baked chicken breast still has 38% fat. Not only do animal foods have more fat, but most of these fats are saturated. Research has shown that saturated fats raise blood cholesterol levels.

A lower-fat, whole-foods diet means fewer calories, since an ounce of fat contains twice as many calories as an ounce of complex carbohydrates. Studies have shown that a diet containing fewer calories can increase health and extend life. It can also help make your perimenopausal transition more pleasant with fewer symptoms.

Decrease Sugar Consumption

Eating a diet high in natural complex carbohydrates tends to be more filling and decreases the desire to consume processed sugars. Lower sugar consumption also decreases overall food intake because foods high in sugar don't satisfy the appetite. As with fat, sugar is a hidden and unwelcome ingredient in many processed foods, especially products labeled low-fat or fat-free. Processed sugars are the greatest offenders to a whole-foods diet. Overindulging in fruit juices can boost your sugar levels to an unnatural high, so drink with moderation.

Eat a Rainbow of Colors and Enjoy More Nutrients!

Eating a greater variety of vegetables also exposes the consumer to, literally, more colorful foods—red beets, chard, yellow squash, red peppers, cabbage. This is more important than you may have imagined. Variations in color are due to various minerals, vitamins, and other nutrients that perform important health-promoting functions in the human body.

Plant foods are richer sources of nutrients than their animal counterparts. Compare wheat germ to round steak. Ounce for ounce, wheat germ contains twice the vitamin B_2, vitamin K, potassium, iron, and copper; three times the vitamin B_6, molybdenum, and selenium; 15 times as much magnesium; and more than 20 times as much vitamin B_1, folate, and inositol. The steak has only three nutrients in greater amounts: B_{12}, chromium, and zinc.

Experience More Food Satisfaction and Less Overeating

Foods such as vegetables, whole grains, and beans that are dense in nutrients and fiber require more eating (chewing) time and result in consumption of fewer calories. Whole foods will satisfy you more quickly, which means you'll eat less. If you are concerned with body image, a whole-foods diet is a responsible way to achieve and/or maintain your ideal weight. In addition, eating less is associated with longevity and optimal health.

Eating Lower on the Food Chain

While it is preferable that a whole-foods diet be as plant based as possible, it may not be necessary to eliminate meats and other animal foods from the diet totally. Today, many kinds of dairy products are lower in fat, and many kinds of animal foods are low in fat. Even so, meats and other animal products should be eaten occasionally rather than as a staple, to add variety to your diet once or twice a week. Always choose the leanest meats possible to cut down on calories, weight gain, and toxic exposure. Alternatively, you can eat more often, but use meat as a flavoring, such as in a vegetable stir-fry, with a few pieces of diced chicken tossed in.

There are many reasons to stick to a more plant-based diet. Important antioxidant nutrients including vitamin C, beta-carotene, vitamin E, and many cancer-fighting substances known as phytochemicals are found in fruits, vegetables, and grains. These antioxidant nutrients are considered the best protection against age- and environmental-related diseases, from dandruff, bad breath, and wrinkling to perimenopausal symptoms, cancer, diabetes, and heart attacks. In many studies, vitamin A has been associated with increased immune response.

The high-fiber content of plant foods helps keep the digestive tract clean by absorbing and eliminating many potentially dangerous toxins. Plant foods also tend to have a lower toxicity than animal foods because they are lower on the food chain and have had less exposure to accumulating toxins.

Medical and scientific evidence points to the benefits of

moving toward a vegetarian-based diet. Dean Ornish, M.D., of the University of California at San Francisco, has demonstrated that a diet free of animal protein, along with exercise and stress-reduction measures, can actually reverse heart disease—the greatest killer of menopausal women. His colleague, James Anderson, M.D., has brought Type II diabetics off of insulin with a vegetarian diet. In 1988, the American Dietetic Association published research showing that a vegetarian lifestyle reduces the risk of heart disease, diabetes, colon cancer, hypertension, obesity, osteoporosis, and diverticular disease.

Part III Healthy Eating: The Basics

Eating is a very personal experience. For some people, it feels like the only aspect of life over which they have control. And it's true: you do have control over what you put in your mouth. So, as you scope out how you relate to food, take a new kind of control and begin eating new foods, healthier foods, less fattening foods. If you follow the tips below for a week, you will, by week's end, realize that the changes don't have to be hard, and that they can afford you delicious flavors and real satisfaction.

- Try not to eat when you're angry or upset, or when you're in a very excited state (even happily so). Wait until you've calmed down or feel better.
- Avoid fast-food restaurants whenever possible. When you're on the go and need a quick bite, remember that there are other options! Rather than heading for the drive-through at your favorite high-fat burger joint, go to a gro-

cery store. Park your car, get out, walk inside, and head for the deli. There you'll find a greater variety, which will enable you to make better choices than that fried burger. It's not important to be perfect; just be aware of what you're eating (and that occasional fast-food hamburger won't kill you, if you really want it). If you travel a lot, seek out healthier "to go" eateries *before* you're starving and need to eat, or pack a lunch. It may take a little while to rearrange your habits, but once you start, you'll find that it's fun to be creative and you'll find ways around unhealthful foods.

- Fill up on fruits and vegetables. Whether for breakfast, lunch, dinner, or snacks, these foods are the way to go. Splurge and try the exotic fruits such as mangos, papayas, kiwis, melons, and hybrid fruits. They're all delicious, sweet, and good for you. Eccentric vegetables such as plantains, various squashes, and different types of mushrooms are fun too. The old standards are also fine. Keep a tray of bite-sized carrots, celery, broccoli, and green and red peppers on hand to answer the need to crunch. And if you want, you can jazz them up with healthy dips such as salsa, yogurt, or Dijon mustard, or toss them in a quick stir-fry. Keep the foods at temperatures you prefer (some people like a really cold orange, others prefer room temperature) and rely on these healthy alternatives especially when craving a snack. Shun those cookies, crackers, and chips, and keep on going back to the natural sweetness of fruit and the crunchy flavors of fresh vegetables.
- Stay away from the unhealthy oils (see page 98). Use nonstick cookware if you need to, or bake, poach, or broil your foods. If you want a little zest, add vinegar, lemon, or spices, especially cardamom, curry, garlic, cinnamon, and ginger, all of which are good immune boosters!

- Eat slowly and ritualistically. Turn off the television. Share a meal with a friend or family members, or, if you're dining alone, make a special place for yourself at the table. Place flowers where you eat. Like music? Put some on before you sit down to eat. Wait until after you eat to read. Take the time to relish and enjoy eating, especially now that you know you're feeding yourself for a healthier life. And try not to scarf your food down. Chew deliberately. Taste it. Explore the flavors. Eating can continue to be a magnificent, comforting experience, one that is indeed in your control.

Of course, this plan isn't easy to follow if you try to make all the changes at once. Instead, try steps out one at a time, see how you like the results, and then jot your feelings down in your journal. While you are adjusting to this new way of looking at food, you're making some lifestyle changes.

There are several shortcuts that can help you in this transition, such as getting a slow cooker to make beans and rice, so there is some staple ready for each day. You can add some fruit or vegetables or tofu and make a unique dish so that you don't get sick of eating the same thing every day. Make fresh vegetable soups that you can use as entrees or side dishes. Explore the many different cuisines of the world for ideas and inspiration. View this as an adventure, an opportunity to do something fun and unique for your heart, body, and mind. Check the Where to Find Help section in the back of this book for a selection of healthy and fun cookbooks.

THE PERILS OF TOO MUCH CAFFEINE

If it tastes and smells so good, can it really be that bad? In the case of caffeine, the answer is yes.

Implicated in everything from hypertension to faulty digestion, excessive caffeine is one of the more potent stressors on the human body. First, caffeinated foods such as teas and coffees come from some of the most pesticide-sprayed crops in the world. Second, there's very little benefit that has ever been derived from any of the caffeine-containing substances and many negative side effects. Third, it interferes with the functions of the liver. Caffeine is a diuretic, so it increases urination, robbing the body of vitamins and minerals contained in the urine—particularly vitamin B and magnesium, which are two nutrients women are often deficient in.

Caffeine has an acidifying effect on the body. Your body tries to correct the acidification by pulling calcium from the bones, so caffeine becomes a causal factor for osteoporosis. It can be particularly hard on perimenopausal women, as it offers your body a false sense of energy and then actually depletes your body of essential energy. If your body doesn't recognize that it's tired, you can't appropriately rest and rejuvenate. It overworks the adrenal glands, making you tired and sluggish.

Other side effects from caffeine include anxiety, nervousness, and irritability, as well as insomnia. Since these are all potential symptoms of perimenopause, it doesn't make sense to seek out a chemical that can exacerbate problems. If you must drink coffee, sodas, or teas, try to reduce the amount. If you can, try mixing your caffeinated beverages with a decaffeinated product, or limit your intake to one serving a day. Be aware though, that decaffeinated beverages are not completely without caffeine.

The Food You Eat

Throughout life, but especially during perimenopause, what you eat affects how you feel and whether your body is being supported. Organic foods are the best choice for your health and well-being. They include all plant foods grown without chemical fertilizers, pesticides, and herbicides, and animals raised on organic feed and not given antibiotics and hormones.

Eating organically helps keep the planet cleaner. Those who grow their plants and livestock organically maintain the purity of the earth's water supply by avoiding the use of poisonous toxins. When buying organic, you also support American farmers working on small family-owned farms.

As often as possible, buy foods that have been produced free of chemicals. It is easy to begin by purchasing organically grown whole grains and beans available in most natural food stores. Organically grown onions and carrots are commonly found in many grocery stores as well.

The label *natural* on nonanimal foods is meant to indicate that the food is healthy and not processed, but it tells you nothing about whether the food was produced with or without the use of chemicals, antibiotics, or hormones. On animal foods, *natural* means only that the animals have been taken off all antibiotics and hormones 15 days before slaughter. Naturally raised animal foods are better than commercially raised animal foods, but when available, choose organic.

Drink!

Our mothers were right when they told us to drink more water. There's really nothing better for your body than good old H_2O. Although the standard eight 8-ounce glasses daily sounds like a lot, it's not once you get in the habit. Our bodies are largely made up of water, so on the most basic level water hydrates the body so that it can perform the basic functions necessary for life. If you're in perimenopause, varying hormone levels can cause your body to work harder, making water even more valuable to your system.

If you drink alcohol or caffeine regularly, you should also

make sure to drink at least eight glasses of water daily—more if you can—since these substances deplete the body of essential nutrients. Be very aware of where your water is coming from. Water that is purified should be your choice, and that doesn't necessarily mean the expensive bottled kind. You can install a water purifier to your kitchen tap, or you can order large bottles to be delivered to your home.

Filling Your Plate

With all the diets and healthy eating plans discussed in the media today, it's hard to know how to fill your plate. Here's an easy formula. For maximum health and vitality, you should be eating 30% to 40% whole grains, 20% to 30% proteins (beans, nuts, seeds, and possibly animal foods), and 40% vegetables and fruit.

This breakdown assures that you will have enough protein, which is in whole grains, beans, nuts, seeds, and vegetables, as well as animal foods. And you'll be getting a lot of vitamins and minerals in all the plant foods.

Eat or Delete

The following is a breakdown of foods that you may want to avoid as well as foods that can boost your energy and help your body efficiently make it through this transitional period.

In General

Delete refined sugars, caffeine and coffee, processed oils, refined white flour, and refined grains

Grains

Eat whole wheat, brown rice, buckwheat, millet, cornmeal, oatmeal, whole-grain pastas

Delete white rice and refined flour (found in white bread, bagels, crackers, cookies)

Beans

Eat navy, black, adzuki, chickpea, lentil, pinto, soybean, kidney

Delete canned baked beans

Vegetables

Eat fresh vegetables, especially yams, winter squash, sweet potatoes, carrots, bok choy, asparagus, Chinese napa cabbage, mushrooms, dark leafy greens (kale, collards, turnip greens), flash-frozen vegetables (without preservatives)

Delete canned vegetables

Fruits

Eat fresh and dried fruits, berries, citrus, black currants, figs, avocados, apples, plantains, cherries, apricots

Delete canned fruit

Raw Nuts and Seeds

Eat almonds, walnuts, chestnuts, hazelnuts, cashews, sunflower, sesame, and pumpkin seeds

Delete commercially roasted nuts and seeds

Fish

Eat baked and broiled salmon, sardines, mackerel, herring, tuna, trout, oysters, shrimp, clams, roe

Delete deep-fried fish and shellfish

Poultry and Meats

Eat chicken, duck, beef, lamb, game, organic liver

Delete fried chicken, luncheon meats, nonorganic liver

Fats and Oils

Eat extra virgin olive oil, flaxseed oil, unsalted butter, unrefined sesame oil

Delete refined and processed oils, margarine, hydrogenated oils

Sweeteners

Eat natural sweeteners such as maple syrup, molasses, rice syrup, barley malt, fruit juice

Delete refined sugars

Beverages

Drink filtered water, fresh juice, grain coffee substitute, herbal tea, green tea

Delete coffee (with and without caffeine), caffeinated teas, alcohol, sodas with phosphates (sugared and diet), sugared drinks

Part IV Eating to Supplement Your Body during Perimenopause and to Reverse Symptoms

Diet matters. You may not like it, and you may not want to change. But if you're serious about your health and want to support yourself through perimenopause, read this section with an open mind. Learn what you can, then adjust your habits so that you feel good about what you eat.

As mentioned in Chapter 3, there is no magic menu for easily navigating through perimenopause. This is why we strongly suggest monitoring your path in your perimenopause journal. Because everyone's body is different, your reaction to different foods and different food combinations will also be different. Observe how you feel, how your digestion and elimination are occurring, and how your energy level is changing. You'll experience a new level of awareness.

Facing What Ails You with Phytoestrogens

While most women experience a wide range of mild to moderate perimenopausal symptoms that can be easily managed with dietary changes, nutrient supplementation, and natural progesterone, there are many others who experience severe symptoms that do not subside easily. These women are generally placed on synthetic hormone protocols and antidepressants largely because their doctors don't know how else to manage symptoms, especially if they are still menstruating and thus aren't officially in menopause.

These extreme symptoms, which most often include hot flashes, night sweats, and bouts of depression, can be associated with wide surges in estrogen levels. As discussed earlier, your perimenopausal symptoms are associated with a state of estrogen dominance. Symptoms worsen if your estrogen level is suddenly magnified, then takes a quick dip again and again. This is where phytoestrogens come in handy.

Phytoestrogens (usually isoflavones, phytosterols, saponins, or lignans) are mild plant estrogens that can alleviate symptoms by performing a delicate balancing act of smoothing out your body's own unique hormone levels. In short, phytoestrogens seek out the imbalances of estrogen and progesterone in your body and then stimulate these hormones if they are too low or help reduce them if they are too high.

While the results of these simple compounds may seem too good to be true, they're not. Many studies have been performed on women from Asian countries who eat a largely plant-based diet, including a great deal of soy products (which contain phytoestrogens and other phytonutrients). The women reported no perimenopausal or menopausal symptoms. However, when these same women began eating a Western diet that was high in animal products, they did begin to report these symptoms.

Some foods high in phytoestrogens include soy, fennel, celery, parsley, clover sprouts, high-lignan flaxseed oil, and nuts and seeds, especially rye.

Other Nutrients for Perimenopausal Women

As scientists begin to discover what foods are good for women, new nutritional stars are making their debut. The nutrients described below play numerous roles in supporting your body during the many changes you'll face in the upcoming transition.

Boron

This mineral helps metabolize calcium and maintain motor skills and mental alertness. It can also mimic and enhance the action of supplemental estrogen. Two large apples, a cup of broccoli, or a handful of nuts supplies about 1 milligram of boron; you should have 1 to 3 milligrams of boron daily.

Essential Fatty Acids

The essential fatty acids included in walnuts, flaxseed oil, dark leafy greens, and fish help prevent perimenopausal symptoms, regulate menstruation, improve the condition of hair, nails, and skin, and help prevent heart disease and cancer. The average healthy adult requires 4 teaspoons of essential oils per day, but if you have perimenopausal symptoms you'll need up to 2 to 3 tablespoons more per day until your symptoms improve. A 4-ounce fillet of salmon provides your day's requirements, as does a large spinach salad.

Special Healing Foods

All whole, natural foods have regenerative and restorative powers. Indeed, meeting the health needs of the body is the aim of a balanced diet. Some foods, however, are unusually rich in nutrients and contain unique chemical components. As mentioned earlier, you should strive toward a balanced diet of 30% to 40% whole grains, 20% to 30% proteins (soy, beans, nuts, seeds, and possibly animal foods), and 40% vegetables and fruit. The following foods should be liberally integrated into your balanced diet as a way of managing your symptoms and boosting immune function.

Garlic

This member of the lily family has well-documented health benefits, including reduction of serum cholesterol and triglycerides, prevention of clot formation, reduction of blood pressure, and enhancement of immune capacity through stimulation of natural killer cell activity. Garlic has sulfur-rich compounds: allin and allicin, chromium, phosphorus, and sulfur-containing amino acids. Raw garlic swallowed in small pieces with water, like tablets, is a great flu remedy, or its cloves can be whole roasted and brushed lightly with oil. If you are worried about bad breath, chew a sprig of parsley.

Ginger

The roots of this reedlike plant contain compounds called gingerols and shogaols that relax the intestinal tract, prevent motion sickness, and relieve nausea and vomiting (especially during pregnancy). Ginger is an excellent source of minerals, especially manganese, which many perimenopausal women are deficient in. Ginger ale can be a delicious bottled form of this food. Buy only natural brands at health food stores and avoid the overprocessed, sugar-sweetened, grocery store brands. Note: Ginger can aggravate problems associated with elevated estrogen levels in women, so don't incorporate large doses of ginger into your diet if you're one of the 30% to 40% of perimenopausal women who are experiencing severe symptoms such as hot flashes.

Blackstrap Molasses

Drop for drop, blackstrap molasses contains more calcium than milk, more iron than beef, and more potassium than bananas. It's easily used as a sugar substitute or eaten in place of jam and jelly.

Yeasts

These single-celled organisms contain high concentrations of B vitamins and many minerals including chromium, one of the key longevity nutrients. Yeasts can be purchased in dried form and sprinkled on top of many foods. Baker's, brewer's, and torula yeast are the three forms of nutritional yeasts most commonly available. Do not eat yeast or yeast products if you have candidiasis, the overgrowth of a naturally occurring fungus *(Candida albicans)* that may occur when the immune system is weakened. (This condition may contribute to other immune deficiency health conditions such as chronic fatigue syndrome.)

Fermented Foods

Cheese, yogurt, buttermilk, sauerkraut, and beer are familiar examples of fermented foods. These foods are processed with enzymes from bacteria, yeasts, and molds that create gradual chemical changes in the structure of the foods. Fermented foods aid in digestion and balance bacterial populations in the gut. They also have a naturally long shelf life and retain their vitamin content much longer than nonfermented foods. Any foods high in fat should be eaten in moderation.

Raw Foods

Although raw foods have a greater risk of contamination by microorganisms than cooked foods, this risk is minimal with high-quality foods and is more than offset by the gain in nutrients and enzymes that would otherwise be lost in cooking. Also, high-fiber raw foods have water-absorbing properties that make them especially effective in absorbing digestive juices from the gastrointestinal tract, thus helping to regulate the digestive process. These benefits are only possible if the raw foods are well chewed.

Raw Juice

There is no better way to get the high-level nutrients from fresh organic vegetables than to run them through a juicer.

The bioflavonoids in the pulp of peppers, for example, will be in the juice along with the vitamin C. Experiment with different combinations such as parsley, spinach, and cucumber; or carrot, celery, and beet. Add fresh garlic and ginger for an immune boost.

Putting It All Together

After reading this chapter, you probably have a good idea of what you need to do. Take a personal inventory of your eating to help you determine the changes you need to make. Don't tackle everything at once. Try things a bit at a time and gauge your reaction.

Begin making changes to a whole-foods diet. Enjoy the freshness of these foods. Integrate phytoestrogenic foods into your new diet. Then supplement your meals with foods that can reverse your perimenopausal symptoms. Again, continually ask yourself how you feel. Chances are, it'll be worlds better.

CHAPTER SEVEN

Use Nutritional and Herbal Supplements to Balance Your Body and Reverse Symptoms

By now, you're fully aware that nutrition is at the heart of your healthy perimenopause. Yet it is very difficult to obtain all the nutrients necessary to maintain good health and create hormonal balance simply by eating a good-quality whole-foods diet. That's where supplementation comes in.

The vitamins and minerals discussed in this chapter are prescribed either for their importance to your overall well-being or as supplemental treatment for imbalances that may be causing your symptoms. Symptoms such as anxiety, insomnia, bloating, nervousness, and irritability are not just signs of hormonal imbalance but are signs of low tissue levels of an essential vitamin or mineral. When you take an oral supplement, the symptoms can often diminish and finally vanish.

Any American walking into a health food store is immediately overwhelmed by the abundance of supplement products. Individual supplements, combinations, prepackaged multi-products—so many of these items promise relief from your symptoms. Yet as you'll see in this chapter, the number of vitamins and minerals that truly restore balance are few. In fact, many women have found relief from the "Quick Fix" shown on page 107.

Herbal remedies that have special significance for perimenopause symptoms are also listed in this chapter. Unlike nutrients, however, which are designed to round out an incomplete dietary program, herbal remedies are designed as a short-term solution. In essence, they are taken to boost or encourage the body to heal or remedy itself.

If you are currently taking nutritional supplements, the information will be easy to digest. If you are new to this way of thinking, helpful tips are presented throughout this chapter that explain how to identify, find, and use quality supplements for your needs.

To help monitor how your symptoms respond to supplements, keep a supplement log using the chart on page 132. Remember to discuss taking supplements with your health care provider.

Part I Nutritional Supplementation

Many women enter perimenopause with a lifetime of nutritional deficiencies caused by an imbalanced diet and a lack of knowledge of their individual needs. Perimenopause is an opportunity to get in touch with your body's needs.

Where to Begin

Every woman can easily integrate supplementation into her lifestyle in the form of a multivitamin. However, multivitamins don't agree with all people, so you shouldn't be discouraged if you find yourself bloating or experiencing indigestion after taking a vitamin. Often the culprits are the B vitamins or vitamin C, which can cause diarrhea in large doses. If a multivitamin doesn't work for you, try taking an antioxidant combination with a multimineral supplement.

Vitamins and minerals come in just about every form imaginable. If you don't like swallowing tablets or capsules, you can also buy vitamins in liquid or powder form. Experiment and find what works best for you.

Choosing a multivitamin can be difficult because there are so many out there, but you can refer to the section that follows for some guidelines. In general, it's best to avoid the supermarket and drugstore vitamins because they tend to have low dosages—check the label. Make sure that if you're taking a tablet, it dissolves. Drop it into a glass of water. If it takes more than 15 minutes to dissolve, find another brand.

THE ONLY QUICK FIX YOU'LL FIND IN THIS BOOK!

Many perimenopausal symptoms, such as mood swings, insomnia, anxiety, dry skin, and water retention, may be alleviated by the following supplement combination:

Vitamin B complex, including 50 to 100 milligrams of vitamin B_6 daily

Vitamin C, 1000 milligrams three times a day

Vitamin E, 400 to 800 international units (IU) daily

Magnesium, 400 to 600 milligrams daily

Evening primrose oil or borage seed oil, 300 milligrams daily

Boost Your Intake of Antioxidants

Antioxidants are important because they fight cell-damaging free radicals, which have been implicated in a number of degenerative conditions, as well as aging. The damage wrought by free radicals is also thought to contribute to discomfort during perimenopause and menopause. Although antioxidants are found in many foods, it is often difficult to achieve the proper levels without supplementation. Here are some guidelines for increasing your antioxidant intake.

Vitamin A and Beta-Carotene

Vitamin A and beta-carotene encompass the carotenoids. These nutrients are crucial for bone formation, among other things, and are found in alfalfa, orange and yellow fruits and vegetables (think color!), fish liver oil, parsley, red peppers, spinach, turnip greens, asparagus, and peaches. Beta-carotene (provitamin A) converts to vitamin A in the bloodstream and is considered by many practitioners to be a better form of the vitamin. In either form, the recommended daily dose of vitamin A for a woman in perimenopause is 5000 IU.

Vitamin C

A diet high in vitamin C can boost the immune system and regulate the body's natural functions. The vitamin is found in citrus fruits, berries, broccoli, beet greens, mangos, onions, papayas, spinach, rose hips, tomatoes, turnip greens, and many green vegetables. The recommended daily dose ranges from 500 to 4000 milligrams, but you can safely take up to 10,000 milligrams daily if you're fighting off a bug. A good test of what your body needs is called bowel tolerance. You can take vitamin C to the point where your stools become loose. At that point, your body is rejecting the excess.

Vitamin D

Building and maintaining strong bones is the main function of vitamin D, which is found in fortified milk, dairy products, fish liver oils, fatty saltwater fish, liver, egg yolks, mushrooms, sunflower seeds, sweet potatoes, vegetable oils, and sprouted seeds. Sunlight also facilitates vitamin D production in the body; only 20 minutes provides your entire day's supply. Most women do not need to supplement with vitamin D (women at risk for osteoporosis may consider 400 to 800 IU daily), since it is one of the nutrients that we get enough of in our daily diets.

Note: Vitamin D should not be taken in supplemental form without calcium, since calcium buffers its severity. Also, it can be toxic in very high doses, so consult your health care practitioner to find the best combination for your needs.

Vitamin E

Often referred to as *tocopherol*, vitamin E is found in avocados, peaches, nuts, seeds, cold-pressed vegetable oils (such as safflower and sunflower), whole-wheat grains and cereals, wheat germ, brown rice, eggs, sweet potatoes, dried prunes, legumes, leafy green vegetables such as spinach, asparagus, peanut butter, and sprouted seeds. Most doctors and practitioners agree that 400 to 800 IU of natural vitamin E daily, taken orally, will help provide the skin and tissues with added moisture and flexibility, including those of the vagina.

Bioflavonoids

These substances are found in plant foods, and they are important because they assist the body in its metabolism of vitamin C and help to build strong capillary walls. We discussed the importance of bioflavonoids in Chapter 6, but here's a review.

Bioflavonoids are available as supplements, but they are also prevalent in soy products, buckwheat, grape and cherry skins, and the inner peel and pulp of citrus fruit. The bioflavonoids are slightly estrogenic and help even out estrogen levels when needed, reducing the body's own synthesis of estrogen or binding with estrogen receptor sites to increase the body's estrogen when low. Asian and African cultures, which feature bioflavonoid-containing foods, have lower rates of breast cancer, very few menopausal symptoms, and fewer perimenopausal symptoms. For the best results, 300 to 500 milligrams should be taken daily.

Minerals for Health

The estrogen dominance that occurs during perimenopause can actually impair the action of cell membranes. The passage of minerals in and out of cells is a delicate balance, and the following minerals are absolutely essential in a supplement program:

Boron, 1 to 5 milligrams daily

Calcium, 500 milligrams daily (take with magnesium for best effect)

Chromium, 200 to 400 micrograms daily

Copper, 1 to 5 milligrams daily

Magnesium, 400 to 600 milligrams daily (at bedtime)

Manganese, 5 to 20 milligrams daily

Selenium, 100 to 200 micrograms daily

Zinc, 15 to 30 milligrams daily

TIPS FOR CHOOSING A NUTRITIONAL SUPPLEMENT

Because supplementation has recently become big business, there are many companies that sell vast lines of products. Unfortunately, some of these companies even sell supplements that contain no active ingredients! For example, in a 1997 analysis of 15 different brands of calcium supplements by the University of Maryland, researchers discovered that the amount found in the samples varied significantly from the amount printed on the label in many of the brands.

How can you make sure you're getting the true ingredients? Obviously, all companies can't be evaluated individually, and new ones keep springing up all the time, but we can offer a few guidelines for being a smart supplement shopper.

1. *You're better off sticking with large, reputable companies.* They have much more at stake than small, unknown companies. Ask your practitioner or retailer for a brief history on the product you are thinking of purchasing.
2. *Don't be a bargain shopper.* There is a wide range of prices, but buying the cheapest product isn't necessarily buying smart. Price should be only one factor in the decision-making process.
3. *Patents count.* If your doctor or practitioner recommends a combination product, check for a patent. A patent is another guarantee of quality for two reasons. First, because rigorous substantiation must be presented to the U.S. patent office before a patent is issued, you can be sure there is good science behind the product. Second, the product manufacturer must ensure that the product being sold contains the exact ingredients specified in the patent, or the manufacturer will risk losing the patent (which typically has cost millions of dollars in research and development). While a patented product is *very likely* to contain what the label claims, remember that the lack of a patent does not necessarily mean another product is inferior.

   Also remember that dietary supplements that exist in nature—for example, zinc—are not patentable. What *is* patentable is the *combination* of zinc and cold lozenges, so you should only buy a combined product if it clearly states "patented" on the label.

4. *Look for the warning label.* If a product makes a health claim, such as "helps maintain healthy, mobile joints and cartilage," then by law the manufacturer is required to run this statement: "These statements have not been evaluated by the Food and Drug Administration. This product is not intended to diagnose, treat, cure, or prevent any disease." If this wording isn't there and the label makes such a health claim, then this company is breaking the law and should be avoided.
5. *Check the product expiration date.* As supplements age, their potency diminishes, so keeping them around for a long time is not a good idea. If you buy large quantities, you may have supplements around for several months. Try to buy supplements with expiration dates at least 9 months in the future.

Part II Herbal Medicine

There are many herbs that can help to balance your hormones and relieve your symptoms. Unlike nutritional supplements or other forms of natural medicine, however, it is not safe to experiment with a wide range of herbal products and dosages to see what works best. "Natural" does not always mean "safe." Mother Nature can be helpful at times and other times dangerous. Wise women will respect that.

So it is important to use herbal supplements with medical supervision. Using this book as a companion guide, your doctor or practitioner can work with you to decide what herbs will work best for your needs and then check to see if any potentially dangerous interactions or reactions may occur. Dosages are provided for general information only. Keep in mind that individual needs may vary.

How Do Herbs Work?

Herbs often have one or more positive effects. Unlike conventional medicines that use one substance to cure or aid one condition, herbs are generally prescribed in a more holistic fashion, with the understanding that all parts of the body work together as a whole. The living cells of plants can be likened to miniature chemical factories. They take in raw materials—carbon dioxide, water, and sunlight—and convert them into useful nutrients. Oxygen is a by-product of this process. Many herbs are rich in compounds that are pharmacologically active—that is, they exert a profound effect on certain animal tissues and organs. Therefore, they can be used as drugs in treating, curing, or preventing disease. A plant may consist of several components including leaves, roots, fruit, flowers, bark, stems, or seeds. Any of these parts may contain the active ingredients that give the plant its medicinal properties.

The herbal pharmacy is a rich one. There are herbs that target specific organ systems and there are herbs that are used as general tonics to promote overall health. For the purposes of this book, we will focus on herbs that boost wellness and reverse perimenopausal symptoms.

There are herbs that soothe pain and inflammation, and still others that ease muscle spasm. Some herbs have a stimulating effect; others have a relaxing effect. Some kill bacteria; others activate the body's own immune system so that it can ward off invading organisms.

Thousands of years ago, when people first began using herbs, they had no idea why herbs worked. All they knew was that a certain plant elicited a desired result. When our ancestors first used foxglove to treat heart failure, they didn't know that this fuchsia-flowered plant contained molecules called glycosides that stimulate heart cells. When mothers in the Middle Ages soothed a scraped knee with a comfrey leaf, they didn't know that the plant's astringent tannins formed a protective surface over the wound, thus promoting healing. When Chinese healers prescribed licorice for arthritis flare-ups, they didn't know it contained saponins, antiinflammatory compounds similar to natural steroid hormones. When the Ancient Egyptians fed garlic to their slaves to keep them healthy, they didn't know it contained volatile oils that fight infection. Many traditional pharmaceuticals were established this way, as well.

Some herbs function in several different ways to alleviate your discomfort during perimenopause. Many of the herbs described in this chapter contain plant hormones (phytohormones), or compounds that stimulate or regulate the body's natural hormone functions.

Thanks to modern laboratory techniques, we now understand how many of these herbs function, adding some scientific detail to a rich legacy of clinical experience. We are able to break down each plant into its basic molecular structure and analyze its extracts. Although we know a great deal more than our ancestors did about how some herbs work, there are still many more that need to be researched. After centuries of firsthand experience, we must still rely heavily on information transmitted through folklore, antique herbals, and word of mouth.

Using Herbs Safely

There's no way to avoid hearing about the healing power of herbal medicine. Yet herbs can be extremely strong medicine, and any effective medicine can have either positive or negative effects. Before taking any herbal medicine, be sure that you know exactly what it does, how to use it, and the possible side effects. Never exceed the recommended dose. As a general rule, few medical problems occur from correctly taking herbal remedies at recommended dosages, but the potential for an allergic reaction is always present. Pregnant women and children should not take herbs unless under the constant care of a skilled medical practitioner.

When getting started, use only one herb at a time, especially if you are using self-care. See if it works and if you experience any side effects. If you're happy with the results, *then* pair the herb with another. If you have a combination of items that are designed to work together, you should still introduce each one individually, trying a new herb no less than 1 week from starting the first one.

Taking the Right Amounts

The amount of herb required for symptom relief may vary from person to person, depending on a wide range of factors (this is why it is so important to consult with a doctor or practitioner). For example, a very small person may require a much smaller dose than a large person. Regardless of age or weight, a person who is highly responsive to medications may require only a small amount of the herb. To accommodate these differences, you should always begin at the low end of the dosage scale and work your way up, to test for adverse reactions. If the herb agrees with you, the dose can be increased to the maximum amount if necessary. If you're finding success at lower dosages, there's absolutely no reason to increase the amount.

Be aware that most herbs should only be taken for a brief period of time for a particular problem and many are not safe for long-term use. Make sure that you learn as much as you can about an herb before you start taking it. Herbs are strong medicine.

Herbs come in a variety of forms, including capsules and tablets, extracts or tinctures, powders, dried herbs, prepared teas, juices, combination products, creams and ointments, essential oils, and personal care products. Most products, however, come in standardized dosages, which makes purchasing and using them much easier. While you should definitely explore the wide range of herbal products available to you, we have chosen to simplify this program by limiting the herbal remedy forms to commercially prepared capsules and tablets, and tinctures.

Many of the more popular herbs are now sold in capsule and tablet form in various potencies. The usual dose, depending on the herb, is 2 to 3 tablets or capsules, taken 2 to 3 times daily. *Always follow the directions provided on the label.*

Extracts or tinctures are liquid herbal products typically prepared by soaking herbs in an alcohol solution. However, there are some new alcohol-free extracts on the market that may be preferable in certain instances, especially for diabetics, pregnant women, children, and others who need to avoid alcohol. The usual dose, depending on the herb, is 10 to 30 drops, 2 to 3 times daily. (This does not include homeopathic tinctures or remedies, which should be used in conjunction with a homeopathic practitioner.)

Part III Homeopathy

Homeopathy is a treatment protocol founded on the belief that *like cures like*. That is, a very small substance of an element can actually trigger your body's systems into healing the condition. Homeopathic remedies are prescribed based on your whole body, not just individual symptoms—although symptoms are often indicative of a body's underlying imbalance, such as perimenopausal symptoms.

Developed 200 years ago by eighteenth-century physician Samuel Hahnemann, classical homeopathy is a natural form of medicine in which extremely dilute preparations of plants, animals, and minerals are given to patients according to the law of similars. This law states that it's possible to cure a sick person of a symptom with a remedy that would cause that same symptom in a healthy person. There more than 2000 homeopathic remedies, but about 100 to 200 are used regularly.

Classical homeopathy embraces a holistic approach to healing, incorporating dietary changes, supplementation, exercise, and mind/body techniques. Acupuncture and some herbal medicines can interfere with homeopathic remedies, however, and some practitioners advise patients not to use these therapies while using homeopathic preparations.

The homeopathic diagnosis consists almost entirely of an interview with the patient that may last from 45 to 120 minutes. The selection of a remedy is dependent on the patient's story and how she tells it.

For women experiencing perimenopausal symptoms, homeopathy is most often used with a more general view of the woman and her transitional situation. A patient will be asked to describe everything about her chief complaints, from menstrual symptoms to the way she feels about this period of her life. The practitioner will try to find out as much as possible about a patient before considering possible remedies.

For the purposes of this book, dosage guidelines are given for mild symptom relief. *Note:* You should consult with a doctor or practitioner before using homeopathy as self-care in conjunction with herbal or nutritional supplementation.

Part IV Treating Your Perimenopausal Symptoms

There is no quick fix for your symptoms. In fact, it may take anywhere from 4 to 6 weeks to see any changes or improvement at all. This doesn't mean that the supplements aren't working. In fact, they are: they are encouraging and stimulating your body to heal itself. And there's no better remedy than that!

The following remedies have been reported to work for other women, but you and your practitioner may adjust the formulations if you need to. Some may work well at first and plateau after a period of time. Don't forget that these remedies are meant to ease the transition between your symptomatic period and your hormone balancing. Once you're back on track, using a quality diet and natural progesterone cream, you'll find that your need for these remedies will diminish.

To make this book a bit easier to follow, we have tried to streamline the protocol by offering a brief list of the best and most effective symptom reversers. In many cases, this will include a multivitamin. If you cannot tolerate multivitamins, you will need to experiment with different supplements and combinations to see what works best for your symptoms without making you feel worse. To determine the best supplement dosages for your needs, consult with your doctor or practitioner.

HERBAL SUPPORT FOR PERIMENOPAUSE

If you're looking for a comprehensive herbal formula to treat more than one symptom, you're in luck: there are many good products out there. The trick is in finding one that works. The most successful formulations for perimenopausal symptoms include the following herbs: *Bupleurum*, milk thistle, barberry or goldenseal, burdock root, yellow dock, and dandelion root.

How to Take Homeopathic Remedies

Remedies come in many forms, but are found most commonly as sugar tablets infused with the remedy. Depending on the form, 15 to 20 granules, or 2 to 3 tablets, constitute a dose. Remedies are commonly available in strengths of 6C, 6X, 30C, or 30X. For purposes describes here, select a 30X or 30C potency.

Take one remedy at a time. Don't eat or drink for fifteen minutes before or after taking the remedy; allow the tablets to dissolve in your mouth before swallowing.

Take one dose daily for three days. Wait one to two weeks to see if there is improvement. Repeat the remedy when and if the improvement stops, taking one dose daily for one to three days. A single dose of 30C can have an effect lasting from a few days to a lifetime, so don't repeat the remedy if it is not needed. If there is no improvement, either the remedy or the potency is incorrect, and a consultation with a homeopath is indicated.

Anxiety and Irritation

Nutritional Supplementation

- Take a good multivitamin/mineral combination containing the dosages recommended earlier in this chapter. A good balance of nutrients will help to prevent or reduce feelings of anxiety. Stress is associated with deficiencies in vitamins B_6 and B_{12}, potassium, vitamin C, zinc, pantothenate, and magnesium, so make sure that these are included.
- If anxiety persists, take a magnesium supplement or a multivitamin with an even higher dose. Low levels of

magnesium can contribute to anxiety and irritation. The usual dosage is 400 to 600 milligrams daily.

- A B-complex vitamin pill is essential, and B_6 has been proven to assist with anxiety. Some multivitamin combinations also include a B-complex component.

Herbal Supplementation

- Products containing black cohosh have been used traditionally to treat anxiety and various studies have shown that this herb does, in fact, have a calming effect. Take one 200-milligram capsule up to three times daily; 1 teaspoon up to three times a day; or 10 to 30 drops of extract (in water or juice) daily.
- Kava kava has been found to have a mildly sedative effect, so it can help with anxiety as well. Take two 200-milligram capsules up to three times daily; 2 teaspoons up to three times a day; or 10 to 50 drops of extract (in water or juice) daily.
- Saint-John's-wort is effective for anxiety related to depression (capsule form). A common folk remedy, the results of this herb were supported in a 1984 study. The usual dosage is one 300-milligram capsule three times daily.
- Valerian is a widely used sedative herb that has antianxiety properties. Take one 300-milligram capsule up to three times daily. Valerian can also be found in herbal teas and is effective if taken 1 hour before bedtime.
- Chamomile is a traditional remedy that has very effective calming properties. Many people find that a cup of good-quality chamomile tea eases anxiety.
- Combinations that include valerian, hops, catnip, skullcap, and passionflower are also effective in treating anxiety. Take as directed.

Homeopathy

- Sepia is a remedy to consider for irritability and fatigue at the time of any hormonal changes, particularly if your irritability is strongest with your family—especially your husband.

Breast Tenderness

Nutritional Supplementation

- Take a good multivitamin/mineral combination containing the dosages recommended earlier in this chapter. A good balance of nutrients will help to prevent or reduce breast tenderness.
- Vitamin E seems to help the hormonal balance and reverse symptoms. You can safely take up to 1000 IU per day.
- Vitamin B_6 acts as a diuretic and may reduce symptoms due to bloating. Usual dosage is up to 300 milligrams per day.
- Evening primrose oil or flaxseed oil capsules alleviate breast tenderness associated with irregular periods. Usual dosage is one 500-milligram capsule three times daily.
- Iodine supplements may also help when little else does. You should have your iodine levels tested before taking any additional iodine.

Herbal Supplementation

- *Vitus agnus* is an overall hormone balancer and may relieve breast tenderness. Take 1 capsule or 1 teaspoon of tincture up to three times daily.
- Red clover helps to balanced stressed adrenals. Take 1 teaspoon of tincture up to three times a day for at least 10 days, especially if you are premenstrual.

- Dandelion leaf and licorice are diuretics that may reduce swelling. For either remedy, take 1 teaspoon of tincture three times daily.
- Chasteberry decoction or tincture (10 to 30 drops in a 6-ounce glass of water).
- Fennel seed and sage tea.
- Marshmallow. The usual dosage is one 200-milligram capsule twice daily.

Homeopathy

- *Calcarea carbonica* is a remedy to consider for sore or swollen breasts of you have one or more of the other *Calcarea* characteristics: chilliness, obesity, perspiration, anxiety, constipation, and fatigue.

Endometriosis

Nutritional Supplementation

- Take a good multivitamin/mineral combination containing the dosages recommended earlier in this chapter. A good balance of nutrients will help support your body.

Herbal Supplementation

- Use an herbal combination that includes cramp bark, licorice root, motherwort, prickly ash, and wild yam. Dosages will vary depending on the combination. Follow instructions on the packaging.

Homeopathy

- *Cimicifuga* is a remedy to consider for endometriosis if your pain consists of cramping with shooting pains across the pelvis from side to side or extending down your thighs.

Fatigue

Nutritional Supplementation

- Take a good multivitamin/mineral combination containing the dosages recommended earlier in this chapter to strengthen your body and fight fatigue.
- You can take up to 50 times the recommended daily allowance (RDA) for some B vitamins, so have your doctor check your levels of B. If you are deficient, you will experience extreme fatigue. B_{12} shots are available to get your levels up and then you should supplement with a good B-complex formula. Folate can be taken, as well. The usual dosage of folate is 400 to 800 micrograms daily.
- Vitamin C, up to 3000 milligrams daily.
- Chromium can raise your energy level by stabilizing blood sugar. Take up to 200 micrograms daily.

Herbal Supplementation

- Dandelion helps detoxify the body, which helps to relieve fatigue. The usual dosage is one 100-milligram capsule three times daily.
- Ginseng boosts stamina and can balance hormones. It's best taken with licorice to boost energy. Take 1 capsule daily. Do not take if pregnant or trying to conceive.
- Peppermint, despite its calming qualities, also fights fatigue. Drink it as a tea up to three times daily (as much as you'd like).

Homeopathy

- Pulsatilla or Sepia may be helpful for hormonally related fatigue. Choose Sepia if you feel irritable, and averse to consolation; choose Pulsatilla if you feel weepy and desire consolation, or if your mood alternates between the two extremes.

Heavy Bleeding

Nutritional Supplementation

- Take a good multivitamin/mineral combination containing the dosages recommended earlier in this chapter.
- Iron supplements, in the amount of 30 to 300 milligrams daily. This is really important, because women who menstruate excessively lose a lot of iron in the menstrual fluid. Conversely, studies have shown that iron deficiency can actually cause heavy bleeding. Make sure to have your iron levels checked before taking iron supplements since iron can be highly toxic. Work closely with your doctor to monitor symptoms.
- Beta-carotene. Supplementing with beta-carotene (provitamin A) will help you replace the lost blood with healthy new blood and may actually decrease your bleeding. The usual dosage is 25,000 to 50,000 IU.
- Vitamin C. Take 500 to 5000 milligrams daily.

Herbal Supplementation

- Dandelion. The usual dosage is one 100-milligram capsule three times daily.
- Lady's mantle. The usual dosage is one 200-milligram capsule three times daily or tincture (10 to 30 drops in a 6-ounce glass of water).
- Yellow dock root. The usual dosage is one 100-milligram capsule three times daily.
- Cinnamon tea.

Homeopathy

- *Belladonna* is considered for heavy bleeding of bright red blood, with or without clots or cramping, particularly if you have a craving for lemonade!

- *Magnesia phosphorica* is useful for cramping that is comforted by bending double or by holding a hot water bottle to your lower abdomen.

Hot Flashes

Nutritional Supplementation

- Take a good multivitamin/mineral combination containing high quantities of B complex and C vitamins, magnesium, and potassium. In fact, many multivitamin products are available that are labeled "for menopausal symptoms" or to treat hot flashes. Check the labels carefully.
- Vitamin E, up to 400 to 800 IU daily, until you see a decrease in the frequency, intensity, and duration of your hot flashes.
- Bioflavonoids can reverse hot flashes since they boost total body immunity, and some even have phytoestrogenic properties. Take 900 milligrams daily.

Herbal Supplementation

- There are many good-quality prepackaged formulas for hot flashes. The best include dong quai, licorice root, chasteberry (vitex), and black cohosh. Dosages vary depending on the combination. Follow instructions on the packaging.
- Dong quai is known for its balancing properties and reversal of hot flashes. Take 1 capsule up to three times daily.

Homeopathy

- *Lachesis* is a remedy for hot flashes associated with feeling generally warm, sleep disturbances, a tendency to loquacity, and an intolerance of "restriction"—whether it's your boss or your new turtleneck sweater!

- Almost any remedy may be useful for hot flashes, when it matches your state in every other way. Hot flashes are really the body's "clue" to the transition and often require a professional consultation to assess your general state. In some cases they may be beneficial; the body working in its own wise way to "heat up" the immune system.

Insomnia

Nutritional Supplementation

- Take a good multivitamin/mineral combination containing the dosages recommended earlier in this chapter.
- Most insomnia that occurs during perimenopause stems from a magnesium deficiency. Use between 400 and 600 milligrams daily.

Homeopathy

- *Nux vomica* is a commonly used remedy for balancing the system and can assist in regulating sleep. Take 1 dose every 6 hours until sleep improves.
- Coffea (coffee keeps you awake, but homeopathic coffee can help you sleep!) is helpful for sleeplessness at the time of menopause when you also have a tendency to get overly excited, from good news as well as bad news.

Irregular Periods

Nutritional Supplementation

- Take a good multivitamin/mineral combination containing the dosages recommended earlier in this chapter.

- Use evening primrose oil or borage seed oil to treat symptoms. The usual dosage is one 500-milligram capsule three times daily.

Herbal Supplementation

- For light and missed periods, look for an herbal formula that includes the following: burdock root, dong quai, false unicorn root, ginger, licorice roots, vitex, Siberian ginseng, and wild yam. (Do not take ginseng if trying to get pregnant.) Dosages vary depending on the combination. Follow instructions on the packaging.
- For frequent periods or spotting between periods, take an herbal formula that includes blue cohosh, burdock root, cinnamon, false unicorn root, ginger, licorice root, motherwort, and red raspberry. Dosages vary depending on the combination. Follow instructions on the packaging.

Homeopathy

- The number of possible variations from the normal cycle is great, and clearly reflects the entire system being off balance. In this situation, consultation with a homeopath is essential to select the correct remedy.

Memory Lapses and Loss of Concentration

Nutritional Supplementation

- Take a good multivitamin/mineral combination containing the dosages recommended earlier in this chapter. A good balance of nutrients will help to prevent or reduce loss of concentration.

Herbal Supplementation

- Dandelion helps to clear the mind (capsule form). The usual dosage is one 100-milligram capsule three times daily.
- Ginkgo biloba can stimulate brain function with no known side effects. The usual dosage is one 40-milligram capsule or tablet three times daily.

Homeopathy

- *Lachesis* may be helpful is memory lapse is associated with hot flashes, heat in general, heavy menses, sleep disturbances, loquacity, and intolerance of any kind of restriction.

Mood Swings

Nutritional Supplementation

- Take a good multivitamin/mineral combination containing the dosages recommended earlier in this chapter. A good balance of nutrients will help to prevent or reduce mood swings.

Herbal Supplementation

- Chasteberry tincture (10 to 30 drops in a 6-ounce glass of water).
- Evening primrose oil. The usual dosage is one 500-milligram capsule three times daily.
- Pantothenic acid. The usual dosage is one 250-milligram capsule three times daily.
- Vitamin C. The usual dosage is 1000 milligrams three times daily.
- Licorice root. The usual dosage is one 100-milligram capsule three times daily.

Homeopathy

- Pulsatilla or Sepia may be helpful for hormonally related mood swings. Choose Sepia if you feel irritable, and averse to consolation; choose Pulsatilla if you feel weepy and desire consolation, or if your mood alternates between the two extremes.

Vaginal Dryness

Nutritional Supplementation

- Take a good multivitamin/mineral combination containing the dosages recommended earlier in this chapter. A good balance of nutrients will help to prevent or reduce dryness.

Herbal Supplementation

- Preparations of the Chinese herb *tang quai* can help to soften and moisten the vagina (applied topically).

Other Supplements for Hormone Balance

Apart from supplements that directly address symptoms, there are others that you can take to help you balance your hormones and foster well-being. Evening primrose oil and borage oil contain essential fatty acids that function as natural anti-inflammatories. Used before and during the onset of PMS-like symptoms, these oils can make you feel better. Take according to the instructions on the bottle, but make sure to look for a brand that gives you the equivalent of 300 milligrams GLA (gamma-linolenic acid) oils daily.

Quercetin is a bioflavonoid that has potent antioxidant and

antiallergy effects. Found in nutritious foods such as green apples and onions, it's being carefully studied for its potential as a heart disease and cancer preventive. Use 250 to 500 milligrams three times a day between meals.

Selenium, elderberry, echinacea, and antioxidants are used to fight colds and flus as well as infections. Take extra selenium (200 micrograms more than recommended in your daily vitamins, two or three times daily with meals), elderberry (which contains powerful antioxidants; follow directions on the container), vitamin C (up to 10,000 milligrams in divided doses in a buffered form), vitamin E (800 IU), and beta-carotene (25,000 IU). This combination of nutrients supports your immune system so that it can more quickly conquer whatever bug has taken hold of you. You can take these supplements when you know your immune system is compromised, such as when you are traveling, when you feel a cold or flu coming on, or when you have a cold or flu. Don't take them at this higher dosage for more than 2 weeks at a time.

Echinacea is an immune-stimulating herb that can be useful when taken at the first signs of cold or flu (follow instructions on the container).

Perimenopausal Skin Care

There is no cause for alarm. Drying skin and wrinkles will not show up overnight. However, just as vaginal tissue is changing, your exterior skin tissues begin to alter during perimenopause. Your supply of collagen, the protein that keeps the skin firm, decreases, possibly linked to a reduction in estrogen levels. The skin becomes less elastic and wrinkles can appear. But as there are various ways to slow vaginal aging, the body's exterior tissues also respond well to smart eating choices and a healthy lifestyle. The oil-soluble vitamins, A and E, nourish skin tissue, and vitamin C is critical for the formation of collagen. Essential fatty acids lubricate the skin, and being well hydrated by drinking plenty of water can restore volume to skin tissue and dispel fine wrinkles. Avoid smoking, which can dry skin tissue.

Emotional Symptoms and Nutrient Deficiencies

Feeling blue or a little anxious? You might just be a bit low on an essential nutrient. The chemical makeup of the brain requires a constant supply of essential nutrients. The following are the most common deficiencies relating to mental and emotional imbalances:

Deficiency	***Symptom***
Vitamin B_3 (niacin)	Insomnia, nervousness, irritability, confusion, depression
Vitamin B_1 (thiamine)	Depression, memory loss, sensitivity to noise, inability to concentrate
Pantothenic acid	Depression, inability to tolerate stress
Vitamin B_{12}	Difficulty remembering, deep depression, severe agitation, manic behavior
Potassium	Nervousness, irritability, mental disorientation
Magnesium	Paranoid psychosis
Calcium	Anxiety, neurosis, fatigue, insomnia

Supplement Log

List of Treatment by Day and Time	*Monday*	*Tuesday*	*Wednesday*	*Thursday*	*Friday*	*Saturday*	*Sunday*
Dandelion for Irritability	10 to 30 drops in water	10 to 30 drops in water	10 to 30 drops in water	10 to 30 drops in water	10 to 30 drops in water	10 to 30 drops in water	10 to 30 drops in water
St.-John's-Wort	300 mg 3 times daily	300 mg 3 times daily	300 mg 3 times daily	300 mg 3 times daily	300 mg 3 times daily	300 mg 3 times daily	300 mg 3 times daily
Magnesium for Anxiety	400 mg 3 times daily	400 mg 3 times daily	400 mg 3 times daily	400 mg 3 times daily	400 mg 3 times daily	400 mg 3 times daily	400 mg 3 times daily

Supplement for Your Future

While supplementation can certainly make you feel better and may even help you emerge from that terrible blanket of symptoms you may be experiencing, remember that no supplement alone can take the place of a good diet, exercise, and self-awareness of your body's needs. You may have ridden through your younger years with little regard to the way you treated your body, but now is the time to reconsider. If you're reading this book, you're already on the right track.

CHAPTER EIGHT

Exercise!

After you've modified your diet and begun supplementation with nutritional and herbal medicine, exercise is the next step in the program. For many women, exercise has solely been a method for burning fat and staying fit. Yet today, we better understand the way that exercise can improve mood, reduce stress, and boost immune function.

Exercise also creates hormonal responses from the body. Aerobic exercise reduces the body's insulin level and elevates the glucagon level. Anaerobic exercising, such as strength training, causes the body to secrete the human growth hormone. This hormone, a builder and repairer of muscle tissue in adults, is the big fat burner. Glucagon promotes vasodilatation, the expansion of blood vessels, so that more nutrient- and oxygen-bearing blood can reach muscle tissue and take away lactic acid when leaving. But fat-burning hormones are not the only ones that respond to exercise. In fact, exercise is one of the healthiest, most effective, and most natural ways to combat depression and stress. This is because exercise releases endorphins, the neurotransmitters that heighten mood.

In fact, many physicians and practitioners have noted how exercise helps to relieve just about every symptom women experience during perimenopause. Although studies haven't proven exactly why it works, clinical results are overwhelming: exercise helps—a lot. Although not yet proven, many doctors believe that because exercise boosts metabolism, it may also help the body better process nutrients. Other factors added to this mix—a better diet, stress-reduction techniques, nutritional and herbal supplements—appear to be more effective when exercise is a component of the overall program.

Why Exercise?

Before we jump into the nuts and bolts of designing your exercise program, let's look at why exercise helps you manage the symptoms experienced during perimenopause and why it's essential for everyone to commit to regular exercise.

Hundreds of studies have proven that exercise is beneficial for both men and women; the young and old; healthy people and those stricken with disease; even those who have never exercised before. In fact, there's also overwhelming evidence that the people who benefit the most from exercise are those who have been sedentary—even their entire lives—then start, and stick to, a moderate exercise routine.

Whether we do something as simple as lifting a grocery bag or as strenuous as running a marathon, we are essentially asking our bodies to produce more energy. And as part of that requirement, our muscular, nervous, cardiovascular, and respiratory systems, as well as our bones, are put to work and asked to produce. The substances they produce, such as oxygen, carbon dioxide, calcium, and nutrients, are of great benefit to our systems. Plus, the energy that's mustered up helps eliminate toxins or other nasty invaders so that our systems stay cleaner.

Some exercises and activities use more muscles than others do, just as some exercises require more stamina than others. But our bodies are like machines in that each organ, muscle, ligament, tendon, joint, limb, and even our flesh is affected by the use of any of the other parts. Our bodies are, in essence, interdependent in the same way that a car doesn't run by the engine alone. Rather, it depends on tires, a steering wheel, and so forth. And if the tire alignment is out, the gas mileage goes down. If there's not enough oil or water, the engine blows up. The car won't run. The same is true of our bodies. So get up and get moving.

The Benefits of Exercise

According to experts at the Stanford Center for Research in Disease Prevention, there are nine benefits to exercise:

1. It improves the health of the cardiovascular system.
2. It helps control weight.
3. It builds lean muscles.
4. It reduces low-density lipoproteins (LDL).
5. It boosts glucose (sugar) metabolism.
6. It lowers blood pressure.
7. It maintains or increases bone density.
8. It improves state of mind.
9. It slows the aging process.

The Legacy of Exercise

These days, it's a well-known fact that regular exercise is beneficial for many different reasons. For people who suffer from perimenopause, it can help battle insomnia, manage stress and anxiety, help regulate breathing patterns and internal body temperature, and boost self-esteem. Exercise can also reduce the risk of:

- Heart disease
- Adult-onset diabetes
- Colon cancer
- Breast cancer
- Falling and subsequent fractures
- High blood pressure
- Obesity
- Depression
- Osteoporosis
- Frailty resulting from age

Given all this, it's clear that when we engage our bodies in activity, we prime ourselves for greater health and longevity.

EXERCISE FIRST, SLEEP BETTER LATER!

Researchers at Stanford and Emory Universities and the University of Oklahoma reported that people who exercised four times a week fell asleep faster at night than their inactive peers did. They studied 43 sedentary but otherwise healthy men and women aged 50 to 76 who had mild to moderate sleeping problems, such as taking longer than 25 minutes to drift off at night and getting only 6 hours of sleep.

The participants were divided into two groups: one engaged in brisk walking and low-impact aerobics four times a week; the other remained inactive. After 16 weeks, those who exercised regularly reported that they fell asleep about 15 minutes faster and slept almost an hour longer than before. Those who did nothing said their sleep patterns were unchanged.

Getting a Jump on Mobility and Exercise

What types of exercise are best for women with perimenopausal symptoms who haven't regularly exercised up until now or aren't really motivated or interested in exercise?

Most people perceive that exercise means more than doing household chores or walking to the end of the sidewalk to pick up the newspaper. If, however, these activities seem strenuous, they may be enough to begin with.

But as time progresses and your commitment to mobility deepens, you'll see there are choices you can make within the very framework of your day that will provide you with even just a few more opportunities to be more active. Perhaps you'll choose to park at the end of a lot and walk farther to the store. Or maybe you'll choose to mow the lawn yourself instead of hiring the kid next door to do it. All these seemingly small choices contribute to a much larger picture of health. They are demonstrations that you won't sit still and let your symptoms get the best of you.

So no matter how insignificant the changes may seem, now is a good time to start recognizing when and how you can make those extra efforts. They will signal to your brain that you are gearing up for the six-step plan, even if that means easing into it one baby step at a time. Remember that the first step always has to come before the second, the second before the third, and so on. And sometimes you'll do the dance of one step forward, two steps back. But that's okay, too. We all have good days and bad days. The most important thing to remember is to have days in which you are choosing more for yourself—more mobility, more activity, more open-minded choices about how to construct a healthier day.

Part I The Seven Types of Fitness

Although a few Olympic athletes know this, few of the rest of us do, so don't feel silly if you don't. And the only reason we want to explain it is so that you'll have more information to work with, thus increasing your innate ability to heal. There are seven types of physical fitness:

1. Strength
2. Aerobic capacity
3. Flexibility
4. Agility and balance
5. Sport specific
6. Power
7. Speed

Since power, speed, and sport-specific fitness have little to do with the kinds of exercise that can be of any initial benefit to your symptoms, we'll let the competitive sport members do their own research on those categories. We'll stick with what can help you and improve your transition through perimenopause.

BE SENSIBLE!

As you think about your goals for fitness, be sure to include common sense in the program. Warm up your muscles and joints before you begin. Stretch your body and joints through all their motions. Slowly increase your activities. If it hurts a lot, don't do it. If it is reasonably comfortable, go ahead.

Strength

The simplest reason to strengthen your muscles is because strong muscles are key to a strong body. Strengthening muscles also increases bone mass, which will benefit you as you enter into menopause by giving you the added advantage against osteoporosis.

A strong muscle is defined by its capacity to exert force through the contractions of muscle fibers. Since the size of the muscle determines its strength, men tend to have the ability to exert more force than women do. Sexual hormones and cultural conditioning also contribute to how much weight a man can bear and a woman cannot. Yet here we're talking about strengthening the muscles that are there, regardless of size, and improving their endurance.

Endurance is measured by the ability of muscles to *repeat* contractions against resistance over a specific period of time. It is also measured by the amount of time you can *sustain* a specific muscle contraction. The more you demand of your muscles to repeat and sustain contractions, the more they will be able to do. The more you demand, the more you stimulate blood flow, which in turn feeds oxygen, nutrients, and enzymes to the muscle. When the muscle is nourished, it wards off fatigue.

There are three basic methods to improve strength and endurance of a muscle:

1. *Isometric force*, which means contracting a muscle and holding it still for several seconds. Lifting a jar of pickles and holding it in the air straight in front of you for at least 6 seconds could do that. The problem with isometric activities is that they only work on isolated muscles. They don't provide a very good overall strengthening and endurance program, but we'll elaborate on that later.
2. *Dynamic or isotonic force*, which means contracting a muscle and moving it from one place to another. That might mean

picking up a shovel with a straight arm, lifting it, rotating your arm in a 90-degree angle, then setting it down. Free weights or weight-bearing exercise machines at gyms provide this kind of strengthening. The more these activities are done, the more resistance you'll be able to lift and move. This type of movement also creates motion with joints. It is excellent for overall toning, especially if the movement uses several different muscles.

3. *Isokinetic force*, in which the speed of the contraction remains constant, but resistance offered by the machine (usually required for this type of contraction) matches the individual's capability throughout the range of motion. This type of conditioning is also good.

Lifting free weights or using muscle-strengthening machines is typically how strengthening and improving endurance occurs most efficiently. But if you're not ready to go to the gym yet, remember the jar of pickles and the shovel!

Bear in mind that if strength is your objective, the number of repetitions you do should remain minimal, while the resistance you use to force the contraction should remain high. If, however, endurance is what you're after, go for more repetitions and less resistance.

Aerobic Capacity

Your ability to keep moving (stamina) while working your muscles is how aerobic capacity is measured. Generally speaking, if the activity you're participating in boosts your heart rate for 15 to 20 minutes, you are engaged in aerobics.

Running, walking, swimming, biking, dancing, rowing, and many more activities test or build your aerobic capabilities. They also promote healthier bones that will support you for many years to come. Aerobic exercise is beneficial because it can help you maintain a healthy weight and reduce stress.

Aerobics and Exercise

From the moment we start to do physical activity, our muscles need more and more fuel. The fuel of choice for low- to moderate-intensity exercise is fat. Aerobic exercise stimulates the release of fat from fat tissues so that the working muscle can burn it. That's why aerobics—or any kind of cardiovascular exercise—facilitates weight loss.

Aerobics is the best type of exercise for an effective cardiovascular workout. When you swim, for example, your heart is pumping blood to the muscles you're working. And the more efficiently your heart is delivering the goods, the longer you'll be able to swim continuously.

Your heart isn't the only organ at work during aerobic activity; your lungs, arteries, capillaries, cells, and veins all contribute to carrying the oxygen, carbon dioxide, and other nutrients to the muscle. They also help eliminate wastes from the muscles. Meanwhile, the muscles you're putting to work rely on glycogen for fuel, which is conveniently stored within the muscles themselves. As long as there's enough fuel and oxygenated blood being sent to the working muscles, you won't feel fatigued. If, however, you exercise beyond the capacity of your muscles to feed off the nutrients, then lactic acid builds up within the muscles and causes fatigue. That's the point at which you feel like you can no longer go on, and exclaim, "Enough!"

You can build up your aerobic endurance and create a change in your physiological structure through four different means:

- *Frequency:* The more often you do it, the more quickly changes will occur.
- *Intensity:* The more intense your workout, the sooner the changes will occur.
- *Time:* The longer you engage in the aerobics, the greater the impact it will have on your body.

- *Type of exercise:* If you swim, you'll use different muscles than if you ride a bike. Cross training, which we'll talk about later, is a good idea, since it ultimately covers most of the muscle groups within your body.

The types of physiological changes you can expect include favorable improvements with:

- Resting heart rate and blood pressure, submaximal exercise heart rate, and blood pressure and body weight
- Body composition (the percentages of the body that are muscle and bone by comparison with body fat)
- Lipoproteins (chemical structures present in the blood that carry fat, proteins, and cholesterol)
- Fat and carbohydrate metabolism (the way the body uses fat and sugar carried in the blood)
- Bone mineralization

Regular aerobic workouts do all that and make you feel better emotionally. That's something worth jumping about!

Flexibility

You're probably already an expert on flexibility . . . or rather inflexibility if you haven't been exercising. And due to the inflexibility, it's easy to strain or sprain the adjoining muscles and stress out other parts of the body that are trying to compensate for the static areas. This is why it is so important to regain flexibility in the places where you have become immobile. Stretching is the best way to improve flexibility, and regardless of your condition, you can start a stretching program today with slow, deliberate moves.

There are three types of stretching of which you should be aware:

1. *Static stretches:* In this stretch, you move the joint to lengthen the muscle and tendons, holding the stretch for 20 to 30 seconds. For example, you could push the palm of one hand down with the palm of your other hand until you feel the muscles and tendons stretch. The longer you hold it there, the more it will "give." Static stretches are safe, as long as you don't push to the point of pain. Over time, these stretches will increase mobility and you'll see a clear difference in your flexibility.
2. *Ballistic stretches:* This kind of stretching is dangerous as it involves bouncing or jerking of the muscles and tendons. You may see runners using ballistic stretches as they bend over and reach for their toes. Their stretches often bounce at the waist. This is not recommended, however, since it can result in injury.
3. *Dynamic stretches:* Refer back to the static stretch of your wrist. You could take that stretch one step further by moving your wrist in slow, careful circles while it is in its most stretched position. There is no bouncing or jerking; rather the full range of motion of the joints is checked while the tendons and muscles are stretched.

An understanding of the importance of stretching has evolved in the past decade, and the bookshelves in most bookstores illustrate that. There is a vast array of information about ways to stretch for specific conditions, types of stretching exercises that improve particular muscles, and so on. Stretching requires no equipment, no fees, nobody else, and can be done just about anywhere.

Agility and Balance

Agility and balance are important qualities for being physically fit since they help keep you on your feet without falling. Measuring agility and balance is slightly more elusive than measuring the other types of fitness. Some people are more coordinated in one activity than another. Standing on one foot may be difficult for you, but chasing after tennis balls might be a cinch.

The important thing to remember here is that maintaining balance and agility is vital for your overall well-being. By designing an exercise program in which you cross train, you can pretty much be guaranteed that your agility and balance will strengthen. Dance, martial arts, yoga, tennis, racquetball, and even badminton engender greater agility, balance, and coordination.

The Stay-at-Home Weight Machine Option

You hate gyms. The YMCA is too far away, or you simply don't want to grunt and moan in front of other people. The answer? Purchase equipment you can use at home. If you're happy using free weights, do that. They're easier to hide, and they'll do the trick. Bigger machines need more consideration.

If you want an exercise machine, you can expect to spend between $200 and $2000. If that's okay by you, look around your house, figure out where it will go (do you want it in front of the television? Looking out a window? In the basement so that it's out of sight?), and then decide what kind of equipment you want.

Do you want to row, climb stairs, or sit on a saddle and pretend to be biking? Or do you like the idea of a cross-country ski machine or treadmill? Be sure to know what you like before making the big purchase. That means trying them out and being honest with yourself about what you'll really do.

Once you know what you want, it's time to ask questions of the merchants who sell the exercise equipment. Does the machine have more gadgets than you need? If so, get the simplified (often less expensive) version. Does it have a heart-monitoring device? Does it have guarantees? What's the resale value? Be sure it feels good to you—for example, that it's not too big or too small. Be sure it doesn't make scary or bothersome noises. Be sure it's made well and that you can get someone to fix it if it breaks down.

Stop and Smell the Roses

If, as part of your exercise program, you spend time outside, remember to notice what's around you. For many, the simple joy of getting outside and observing life is satisfying. The exercise just becomes icing on the cake.

The next time you venture out, look up. Notice the sky. Is it a deep blue or a pale soft blue? Are there clouds? Big thunderheads or small wispy ones that look like an artist's brush stroke? Do you see any birds? What kinds of trees surround you? Do you pass by flowers? Notice their colors? Touch them to feel their silky petals? Maybe today, stop and smell them twice as long.

Part II Planning a Regular Cardiovascular Program

Of the four types of fitness already described, aerobic exercise is the most difficult form of exercising for individuals who haven't exercised before or who are returning to exercise. Most people associate aerobic workouts with extreme exertion and misery. Yet it doesn't have to be that way. Ease yourself slowly into an aerobic program and see how you feel. The three most popular forms of aerobic exercise are discussed next with some tips for making them more effective and enjoyable.

Swimming

You can make some real changes in your health care by developing a regular swimming routine. And you don't have to get bored, either, because there are several options for achieving and maintaining fitness for water lovers.

Chances are you don't have a pool in your backyard, but there are probably health clubs, YMCAs or YWCAs, hospitals, and municipal facilities nearby that do. As mentioned earlier, you'll need to find out what times are available for free swimming, as well as the temperature of the water and any classes available.

If laps are what you're after, take your time getting acquainted with the water, and be sure you breathe efficiently. Consult an instructor to help you get your form down. Use a kick board if you don't have the upper body strength you need to carry you confidently. And check out an inner tube for around your waist if you want to remain stationary but still work those hips and knees. There are other devices that can help you reach your goals. Just shop around a little and you'll be amazed at what's out there.

Laps are wonderful, but so are water aerobics classes, or even self-directed sessions of running or walking in the pool. Your routine can be as simple as walking back and forth between the shallow ends of the pool, or running as far as you can until your reach the deep end, then breaking out into a freestyle, sidestroke, or backstroke swim. No matter what you do in the water, it's easier than on land, since there's so little pressure against your joints and muscles.

Even though some people don't think swimming is as good a workout as walking, there's still evidence that those who swim have thicker bones than people who don't exercise at all. That says a lot for the sport, but what will really speak to you is how much better you feel after doing water sports, and how quickly they can improve your flexibility.

If you're new to swimming and somewhat tenuous about it, start slowly by entering the shallow end and doing range-of-motion exercises with your lower extremities. You'll probably find it very enjoyable, and before you know it, you'll be going into deeper water. Finally, you might be in water to your neck while you freely walk, run, or dance around the pool. Your time in the water doesn't have to be structured, but like all aerobics, it does need to be constant in order to get your heart rate up and strengthen those muscles.

Start slowly and at a pace that suits you, but shoot for a good 35-minute routine 3 days a week. It may take a month for you to work up to this, or a year. You're not competing, so it doesn't matter.

Be careful when you get in and out of the pool, making sure to take your time and walk gingerly on the wet walks that surround the water. You will feel heavy when out of the water and it may take a minute to get steady on your feet.

Bicycling

Getting on a bike and cruising around is plain old fun. You cover more ground than walking, and it provides great opportunities to strengthen leg muscles and lubricate those knees.

If you're attracted to biking but don't have a bike, or if the one you have is rusted and mice have eaten away at the tires, consider buying a new one. Mountain bikes have fat, stubby tires that are less inclined to go flat from sharp rocks or road debris, and they provide more stability than bikes with skinny tires. You can get a good one for about $200, but there are models that cost less. Also, used bikes are always around and are typically a good bargain.

If it's been a while, you may not be used to hand brakes or

all the gears that they come with these days. After a few minutes of riding around, you'll probably feel just fine about both. The multiple-gearing system is a bit more complicated than the brakes. Ask the sales clerk for a detailed explanation of how they work, then play around with them on flat land. You'll quickly discover how the gears enable you to pedal really fast and hard on flat land and fairly easily up steep inclines. Pretty soon, you'll be planning a trip to the mountains so that you can conquer a few hills and race down the opposite side.

Helmets are a must. Don't skimp on quality, since a helmet can save your life. Ask a knowledgeable sales clerk about the best brand and for advice on how to ensure a proper fit.

Water cages and lightweight water bottles that fit snugly into the cages are also a must. They are typically right under the handlebars for easy access while you're riding.

Other equipment is available that can help your ride be more efficient or comfortable. Biking gloves cushion your palms from the weight you'll distribute as you lean on the handlebars. Biking shorts are specially padded in the crotch to ease the stress there. And you can attach toe clips to the pedals so that you use energy more efficiently while pumping. You can buy a bike rack for your car so that you don't have to ride your bike through traffic to get to the less congested bike path or road of choice. But all of these things are optional and not critical to a good workout.

Once you've got the perfect bike and bought whatever gear you're after, take it for a spin. As always, take it easy your first day out. If one lap around the block is all you can manage, that's fine. However, if you're feeling pretty comfortable, try for two or three. Remember that if you're not doing a loop, you'll have to turn around and go back as far as you've come. So don't exhaust yourself before turning around. As your body grows accustomed to the routine, you can work your way to that 30-minute goal 3 days a week.

Aerobics Classes

Just about any fitness center or gym in the country offers a grand array of aerobics classes from jazzercise to step classes to water aerobics. Since we've already discussed water aerobics, let's focus now on landlubber classes.

Once again, common sense has to come into play here. Think too about your special needs. If you're attracted to a jazzercise class but haven't exercised in a while, look for an introductory class that may teach you some of the basic routines and break you into it slowly.

Contact the instructor of the class you want to take. And, of course, it doesn't have to be one offered at the gym. Aerobics is a generic term that covers anything that makes you move enough to increase your heart rate. So if you find out about a dance class—whether it's ballroom, jitterbugging, country line dancing, modern or folk dancing—it qualifies as aerobics, too. In any case, since you have special needs, it's important to speak to the instructor to find out exactly how strenuous the class is and determine if you can do it comfortably. If you think you can, call your doctor and make sure there's no objection from that end.

Aerobics classes can be low impact (which is probably where you want to start), moderately difficult, or high impact (which is for those who seem stronger and fitter than the rest of the human race). But don't fool yourself—they can encompass nonstop movement for up to 90 minutes. It might be wise to observe a class first, then determine if it's what you want. And part of determining that is to see if it looks like fun and like something you *want* to do. Remember that there's no reason to do these classes if you're going to resent every skip, jump, and kick.

If you're not sure about how the class could affect you, remember that you can do it at your own pace. You can take breaks even when others keep moving. You can (and should) take water breaks. You can tailor the workout to meet your needs as long as you've discussed it with the instructor beforehand.

The beauty of aerobics classes is that they can bring some real fun into your exercise routine. They expose you to a group of people who can extend into your social circle. They promote range of motion, strengthening, and cardiovascular activities, all of which you need to loosen those joints and pump up those muscles. All that adds up to a good time with spirits lifted and plenty of good movement for your body.

Don't forget to wear good aerobic shoes for classes at the gym, and if you're out dancing, be sure the shoes you wear are appropriate. High heels are discouraged. Visit your local shoe store and check out the cushioned-soled shoes with a more formal appearance. There are ways to look attractive and be comfortable and safe, too. You are the judge of your own capabilities, so work with your body, enjoy yourself, and aim for that 35-minute marker.

The Right Way to a Good Exercise Program

Following the guidelines in this section will make your exercise routine enjoyable, effective, and easy. So read on, take notes, and keep breathing!

Consult Your Physician

Once you've designed your fitness plan, the very first thing you need to do is call your doctor and let him or her know what you have in mind. Getting injured is not on our "To Do" list. Discuss your plans and listen to whatever advice is given to you, as well as to your own intuition.

Read Over Your Goals

Read the list of goals in your journal each day before you exercise. If they suddenly seem unrealistic or too simplistic, change them. But start each routine by first reading and affirming that those are your goals and that you will reach them.

Wear Sensible Clothes

If it's hot out and you're going walking, wear light, breathable clothes. If there's been a nice snowfall and you're setting out for a cross-country ski trip, take appropriate layers of clothing so that you can bundle up if the wind whips up or peel off a layer if the sun is hot. There's often no better excuse *not* to exercise than physical discomfort from inappropriate clothing.

Choose Activities You Enjoy

There's no reason to swim if you can't bear to get wet. Forget riding a bike if you're wobbly on the saddle. It may take some experimenting, but there are lots of options, so choose something you like to do.

Be Comfortable with the Conditions

If you're a swimmer, be sure the temperature at the pool you visit will remain constant, and that you like it. Also, make sure the hours a facility is open match your schedule. As a bicyclist, make sure traffic, rain, and an occasional flat tire don't bother you. If you decide aerobics classes are fun, take the time to interview the instructor, explaining your special needs, and be sure you're in the right hands.

Each type of exercise has its disadvantages. Be honest with yourself about what they are and how they might impact you. Your commitment is key. Don't let the little things bring you down.

Choose the Best Time for Your Routine

You like to sleep late and wake up leisurely with a cup of coffee and the morning paper. Fine, but remember that the day will progress and with it will come a thousand distractions or reasons why you just can't get to your routine. Look carefully at your habits, your schedule, and the demands your routine places on you (for example, you probably want to walk while it's still light outside) and commit to the times of day you will exercise. That can change if necessary, but don't weasel out of it!

Wear or Use Safety Gear

Wearing a helmet while bicycling isn't just for kids. The majority of bike-related deaths occur because the rider wasn't wearing a helmet. If you swim and have sensitive eyes, buy some water goggles. Who cares if you look like a raccoon! And while you're at it, don't hesitate to use devices that might help you along, whether it's a kickboard, an inner tube, or rubber shoes. You're not competing for fashion awards. You're just getting healthier!

Get Professional Instruction

You may think you're lifting those weights just right, but suddenly you have a muscle cramp. What good are toe clips on a bike? How come some people never get winded when they swim whereas others gasp for air?

Whether you decide to work out with free weights or machines, ride a bike, swim, or even walk, it would be wise to get a few hours of advice from a professional trainer. Sometimes even the slightest adjustment can give way to better results.

Cross Train

You like to walk, it's aerobic, and everyone knows it's good for you. So why bother with those heavy, cumbersome weights? Because if you only do one kind of exercise, your muscles won't tone evenly, which can cause biochemical or structural imbalances in your body. Plus, you're going for overall fitness here.

Cross training also keeps you from being bored. If you walk twice a week, ride a bike twice a week, and work out with weights twice a week, you'll not only look and feel better, you'll be more inclined to stick with the program because it won't become tedious.

Determine What, How Often, and When

You can get plenty of advice on what exercises are best for your physical condition, but only you know what you'll actually do. Remember to choose activities you enjoy. Also, be honest with yourself about how often you'll really do them. If you know you simply won't do a 4-day program, then design your program with an honest assessment of how often you will commit to it. The same holds true of when you do your exercises. You're in command here, so be honest, maybe consider striving for 10% more than what you're comfortable with, and see how it all shakes down. But don't fool yourself. If you discover that you actually feel better after a few workouts (surprise!), change your mind and commit to more.

Be Consistent

You could set yourself up for injury if you do your exercises only occasionally. And you certainly won't benefit in the ways we're suggesting. It's essential that you are consistent.

Always Warm Up First

Start by stretching. Then walk, bike ride, swim, or whatever at an easy, gentle pace as part of your warm-up. Your entire warm-up should last between 10 and 15 minutes. It should increase your pulse to 50% to 60% of your maximum heart rate (more on that later).

Don't take warming up lightly. It's necessary for:

- Reducing the risk of abnormal heartbeats
- The appropriate amount of oxygen to be sent to the muscles, which occurs through gradual loosening of them
- Improved range of motion and balanced coordination
- A gentle transition from inactivity to moderate or strenuous activity
- Preventing injuries

Listen to Your Body

Listening to your body isn't as goofy as it sounds. How do you know when you're hungry? When you have to go to the bathroom? When you're sleepy? You may have spent your whole life unaware that your body communicates to you every day—and not only about the need for food, the bathroom, and sleep! Now is the time to listen.

As you exercise, pay close attention to what's going on inside of your body. You don't need to feel extreme pain, so if you do, stop. If you feel mild pain, is it because your muscle isn't used to the exertion, or is it because you're pulling on it the wrong way? With each step you take, each city block you cycle around, each weight you lift, check in with yourself. Have you had enough? Can you do another lap?

Listen closely and before you know it your body will wake you up in the morning with very clear messages about what it needs for the day. Maybe it longs for the kind of workout that water aerobics provide. Or maybe you feel it wanting to push against something like a weight machine. Maybe it's saying it needs a rest! You may not always be able to accommodate what it communicates to you, but at least you will have established dialogue!

Start Slowly

Begin your exercise program slowly and carefully. If you do more than your body can handle, you could get hurt, you won't enjoy it, and you certainly won't want to do it again.

If starting slowly means doing a total of three repetitions with free weights, then so be it. If it means swimming for 2 minutes, then celebrate those 2 minutes! If it means walking from one end of the grocery store to the other, be glad of it! The only judge who can condemn you for not doing more is yourself. The only judge of how much you can really do is also yourself. Make friends with that judge by knowing that you need to go slowly and easily at first. But don't cheat yourself out of more if you can handle it.

Condition Yourself for the Next Step in 3-Week Cycles

Think back through your life. What were the most worthwhile endeavors you accomplished? Did they happen overnight? Chances are, they did not. Nor will getting fit.

Once you start your routine, and if it feels right, stick with it for 3 weeks. Then evaluate whether you can increase your repetitions, cycle another mile, or walk another few blocks. But stick with 3-week increments because it takes about that long to reap the full benefits of any given routine. If, however, at the end of the 3-week period you aren't ready to do more, don't sweat it! Give it another 3 weeks and then decide what's next.

Alternate How Hard You Work Out

Some days, for reasons that may or may not be clear, you might feel like a truck flattened you. Lighten up your routine on those days. Other days, you may think you're Superman or Wonder Woman in the flesh! Go for it! See how much you can do without overdoing it and give yourself a pat on the back or buy yourself a reward.

Even if you don't experience these extremes, it's wise to alternate the intensity of the workout so that you get to know your limits. Observe what happens on both a physical and a psychological level. You might learn something new about your physical prowess or how your mind works for you or against you as your body pushes.

Keep Yourself Hydrated

Drinking water or sports drinks before, during, and after you exercise keeps your potassium and sodium levels in check. Those are the things you sweat out—up to two quarts in an hour!—when you exert yourself, and they're important to replace. Here are some guidelines to staying hydrated:

- Drink even when you are not thirsty.
- Weigh yourself before and after exercise. Drink 1 pint (2 cups) of liquid for each pound you have lost.
- Drink at least 1 cup of water one half hour before exercising.
- Don't drink or eat anything sugary for 2 hours before exercising.
- Drink 3 to 6 ounces of fluid every 15 to 20 minutes during exercise that lasts longer than 30 minutes. Do this even if you're exercising in a cool room and don't feel yourself sweating or don't feel thirsty. If you wait until you are thirsty, you are already dehydrated.

- Drink cool fluids. They hydrate the body faster than warm or ice-cold beverages.

Keep Breathing

That's the best advice. Most exercises will work more efficiently if you breathe properly and you also want to encourage your heart to pump adequate amounts of oxygen to your muscles. What does that mean? It depends on what you're doing. Clearly, if you're swimming, your breathing patterns will differ from when you're riding a bike. As a general rule of thumb, when working with weights, exhale when you're pushing or lifting and inhale when you relax or release. Be sure to consult with the professional you work with about the best way to breathe during your exercise of choice.

Monitor Your Heart Rate

According to the American Heart Association, you need to exercise for 30 to 60 minutes three to four times per week so that you can reap the benefits, especially for the heart. If you exercise more than four times per week, it will increase those benefits. To do that, however, you need to increase your heart rate to 50% to 65%. Keep in mind, though, that intense aerobic exercises may be something you have to work toward. If you're just beginning your exercise program, read the following information knowing that you will eventually be able to attain these goals.

To estimate how to achieve 50% to 65% of your maximum heart rate, make the following calculations:

- Subtract your age from 220. That amount equals your maximum heart rate.
- Multiply that figure times 50%. That equals the lowest number of heartbeats you should reach while exercising.

- Multiply your maximum heart rate by 65%. That equals the highest number of heartbeats you should reach while exercising.

For example, if you are 40 years old, the calculation is as follows:

220 – 40 = 180

180 × 50% = 90 (beats per minute for the low end)

180 × 65% = 117 (beats per minute for the high end)

To achieve the benefits of exercise, your heart rate will have to be at least 90 beats per minute but should not exceed 117 beats per minute. Check your pulse after 10 minutes of exercise to establish your heart rate. If it is below 90 beats per minute, you need to work a bit harder. If it exceeds 117 beats per minute, you need to ease up.

Another way to determine if you're exercising hard enough, or too hard, is by checking your breathing. If, while you bicycle or walk, you are comfortable and can talk with ease, you're not pushing hard enough. Pick up the pace. If, on the other hand, you are gasping and unable to talk at all, you're pushing too hard. If you're breathing deeply but can speak in short sentences, you're probably right where you need to be.

Check your heart rate every 10 minutes or so during your workout and then after you've finished. This will enable you to monitor your progress and determine your next steps.

Cool Down

Few people know that cooling down is even more important than warming up. It enables your pulse to return to normal at a gradual pace. If you don't cool down, it can cause your heart to beat too quickly, which can result in a heart attack or irregular heartbeats. Cooling down also prevents blood from pooling in your legs, which can lead to dizziness, blackouts, and disorientation. Simple stretches after your workout will keep your muscles from cramping, getting stiff, or becoming sore. Do the same exercises to cool down that you do to warm up. Start the cool-down at a slower pace and follow with a series of stretches.

Keep a Record of Your Workout, and Give Yourself Credit

Even if you had a crummy workout and you felt like a complete slug, record what you did in your workout log below and give yourself credit for what you accomplished. If you did only one lap in the pool or three blocks on the bike, write it down. You did it, even if it didn't match up to your expectation, and in the long run it too will contribute to your feeling better, maintaining a healthy weight, and improving your state of mind.

If you had a great day, record that too, and acknowledge yourself for attaining or exceeding your goals. Persistence, an open mind, and a willingness to exercise even if you didn't feel like it has brought you to this point. Congratulate yourself. Reward yourself by buying flowers, going to a movie, or calling a loved one and sharing the good news. Remind yourself of how great you are!

The Next Step

Now that you've integrated a workout program into your life, here are a few suggestions to modify your workout chart:

- Increase your workout days from 3 to 4 or even 5 days a week.

Workout Log

	Monday	*Tuesday*	*Wednesday*	*Thursday*	*Friday*	*Saturday*	*Sunday*
Range of Motion							
Stretching							
Weight Training							
Cardio-vascular							

- Increase your time with each exercise. Begin by adding 10 minutes, then maybe another 10 minutes.
- Stagger your workouts. Maybe do cardiovascular one day and weight training the next and yoga on the weekends. Just don't forget to stretch.

CHAPTER NINE

Use Mind/Body Medicine

Before we discuss scientific explanations of how your mind can improve the symptoms your body is manifesting during perimenopause, let's first define what we mean by *healing.* Even though the emphasis of this book is on the multitreatment way you can improve or eliminate your perimenopausal symptoms, it's important to realize how your physical, mental, emotional, and even spiritual life is intertwined—either working in unison or at odds to make up the overall state of your well-being. It's referred to as the mind/body connection.

If we define *fitness* in physical terms only, then we're dismissing some critical influences that can either support you in obtaining and maintaining relief from your symptoms or keep you from experiencing any relief at all. The influences include how you feel about yourself, the world, your state of physical health, and what you do to take care of yourself.

If, for example, you are depressed because your body is manifesting these different symptoms and you're feeling bitter and resentful that it has limited your activities, then you may indeed read the book, but you might be skeptical about the effects that this information could actually have. Or, you might give this protocol a try, but if you don't see quick results you may quit.

Maybe you're not upset about your condition. Maybe you're excited that the first few steps have already shown improvement in your life, and you now feel energized and ready to commit to the next step. The activities you'll learn about in this chapter will help you do just that.

Deepak Chopra, M.D., is a well-known pioneer of the mind/body connection and has sold millions of books explaining this new medical science. He believes that:

> The essential foundation of mind-body medicine is the recognition that for every experience in the mind, there is a corresponding change in the physiology and biochemistry of our body. We have a vast internal pharmacy that can be accessed through conscious choices we make in our lives. A key tenet of mind-body medicine is that health is not the mere absence of disease. Rather, it is the dynamic integration of our environment, body, mind, and spirit.
>
> Reducing stress through meditation techniques, improving vitality through balanced nutrition, and developing flexibility, energy, and endurance through yoga and exercise are a few of the basic approaches of mind-body medicine, which have demonstrable health enhancing effects. Herbal medicine, massage, sound, color, movement, and aromatherapy are other tools of mind-body medicine that can advance mental and physical well being, and you should look into. Mind-body medicine offers new possibilities for promoting and improving health through natural approaches that stimulate our body's intrinsic healing system. (1990, p. 212)

Mind over Matter

Western medicine has made extraordinary advances over the course of the twentieth century. Central to this progress is the scientific method. By attacking disease and illness with the powerful weapon of rational empiricism, the medical community has won many wars.

But the battle has not been without its casualties. One of these is an awareness of the inextricable connection between the mind and the body. For most doctors, health is simply a matter of body parts functioning properly. When they don't, the mighty arsenal of medications is called on to repair the problem. If these fail to work, even more aggressive action in the form of surgery is pursued.

Certainly drugs and surgical procedures are often necessary to cure illness and injury. But lost in the shuffle is the role that the mind, as well as the spirit, can play in the healing process. In Eastern societies as well as indigenous cultures in the West, the link between physical and mental well-being has always been clear. Meditation, religion, hypnosis, and yoga play a key role in maintaining or restoring health.

Until recently, this integrationist approach was largely ridiculed by Western physicians as primitive superstition. But over the last few decades, growing scientific and public interest has led to the rapid evolution of a new field: mind/body medicine.

Armed with studies demonstrating the relationship between physical health and such variables as mood, attitude, and belief, pioneering researchers are now pushing the heretofore rigid boundaries of allopathic medicine. Do people with a positive attitude stand a better chance of recovering from sickness? Can depression weaken the immune system, leading to physical illness? What contributions can meditation and relaxation therapies make to the healing process? These are the questions being asked and answered by advocates of mind/body medicine.

HANDS-ON HEALING

While constructing your program for optimum health, consider getting a regular massage. Not only is it relaxing and rejuvenating, but it also invigorates muscles, tendons, and ligaments and motivates the body's internal systems. After getting caught up in the demands of everyday life, massage may be the only time you can afford to completely relax, contemplate, and be nurtured.

Some people say they can't afford regular massages. Even so, if massage not only benefits your body but can also help relieve anxiety and depression, as well as make you more aware of your body and what it needs to be healthy, doesn't it make sense to think of massage as an investment in yourself?

Principles of Mind/Body Medicine

Individuality

Conventional medicine tends to lump everyone together in its approach to diagnosis and treatment, offering treatments based entirely on clinical diagnosis. In mind/body medicine, each person is seen as unique, with multiple factors that influence his or her health. This thinking alters both diagnosis and treatment, in that numerous variables may be responsible for a person's illness.

Stress

Mind/body medicine recognizes mental and emotional stress as a significant factor in physical well-being. Operating on the principle that stress can lead to sickness, mind/body medicine seeks to reduce stress through various therapies.

Responsibility

For health to be restored, the patient must take an active role in the healing process. Participation has been shown to aid recovery and decrease fear and depression associated with serious illness.

Self-Healing

If given proper support, the body will tend toward health. Conversely, health will be negatively impacted if the patient does not believe in her healing path or feels powerless to contribute to the healing process.

Patient–Practitioner Relationship

A positive relationship built on trust between patient and practitioner can strongly influence the healing process. Negative, discouraging statements from a doctor may inhibit recovery, as can a relationship that empowers the practitioner and treats the patient as a mindless body.

Multifactorial Approach

Mind/body medicine sees health as the by-product of numerous influences, including genetics, family, socioeconomics, diet, exercise, social support, attitude, and spiritual practices.

Energy Fields

The vital interrelationships between the body's many energy fields can facilitate healing. Discouraging or inhibiting this natural process can be detrimental to the body's inherent energy flow.

Breaking the Stress Cycle: Mind/Body Remedies for Relaxation and Symptom Reversal

It's well documented that physical exercise can do wonders for emotional health. But can the mind really help heal the body?

The answer is a resounding yes, as evidenced in the booming field of mind/body medicine. Through the work and writings of such high-profile visionaries as Norman Cousins and Deepak Chopra, the Western world has begun to understand what peoples in the East have known for centuries: that physical health cannot be separated from psychological and emotional well-being.

Until the 1980s, most doctors tended to regard health as a matter of simple biology. If anything interfered with the body's proper functioning, a drug was pulled off the shelf or a patient was referred to a surgeon.

Of course, medication and surgical procedures are essential in the treatment of illness. But there's a growing realization among health care practitioners that the mind can be a potent force as well in the healing process. This awareness is due in large part to the shrinking nature of global society. As the world's cultures have become more enmeshed, we have started to seek out the healing traditions of societies in which the interconnection between mind and body is taken for granted. For much of the world, practices such as meditation and relaxation are considered essential to basic health. This integrationist approach, once dismissed in the West, is now the focus of intense public as well as scientific interest.

The research community has put significant resources into this new frontier. Prestigious academic institutions such as Stanford University, the University of Massachusetts, and Harvard University have created mind/body programs, studying everything from the chemistry of emotions to the effect of stress reduction on cardiovascular health. Since the 1980s, numerous studies have substantiated long-held beliefs about the relationship between physical health and such factors as stress and depression. In so doing, they have given widespread legitimacy to an array of mind/body techniques that are helping change the face of medicine.

Creative Visualization

Just before you actually begin warming up and prior to subjecting yourself to a public arena (for example, the swimming pool, gym, yoga or aerobics class), find a quiet place and lie down for 5 minutes. (If you need to drive somewhere to work out, do this before you leave your house.)

Get comfortable. Relax your body as deeply as you can. If playing music helps you to relax, put it on. Close your eyes and envision each limb of your body as relaxed and pain-free. Then imagine yourself in the workout in which you are about to partake. Watch yourself warming up, only maybe in your mind's eye you'll be able to stretch just a little bit further than you can in real life. Then see yourself doing the main activity, for example, swimming. Watch yourself immerse into the water. That may be through diving, jumping, or easing in via the pool stairs. See yourself smile as you recognize the weightlessness you feel in the water. Then picture yourself swimming with ease and grace. See your joints moving and all that nutritious synovial fluid pumping in and out as you kick your legs. Feel the strength you are building in your muscles. Watch yourself reach the end of the first lap and feel the increased beat of your heart. Listen to your breathing as it has deepened, but notice you are not gasping. Watch yourself through several laps, all the while recognizing how beautiful you look and feel in the water. Then watch yourself get out of the pool, dry off, and take a deep breath that refreshes you and brings you back into your present reality. Now take a few deep breaths.

If it's hard for you to imagine yourself and keep control of the thoughts in your mind's eye, then simply focus on relaxing your body and repeat your affirmations over and over. Squeeze in an image of yourself whenever you can: remember what you looked like and felt like at your healthiest, or picture what you would like to look and feel like in a year.

When you take 5 minutes before your workout and visualize

these things, you are sending messages to your body and unconscious mind that these states are what you want and that they can be achieved. It will prepare you for your workout and represent the routine as a pleasant, rewarding experience. If you find exercise especially difficult or unpleasant, creative visualization may help you. Do it every time you work out. It does work and it will make a positive difference.

Emotional Healing

Joan Borysenko, Ph.D., a pioneer in the field of mind/body medicine, adheres to a simple philosophy: "Whenever we are isolated, we're stressed, and when we are connected, we are more likely to be healthy." For Dr. Borysenko, this belief translates into a need for high self-esteem and good social support. "Health varies with relationships," she says. "When your relationship is right—that is, you have right relationship to self and are able to be authentic, to have figured out what your values are, what are the most important things to you, and then live your outer life according to those inner values—then you are in good relationship to self. When you do that, then you have a better chance of being in good relationship to others and to really establish bonds of intimate trust with other people."

The third level of right relationship, says Borysenko, is people's philosophic relationship to God or life or the source of being—"whether, in Einstein's terms, they think the universe is a friendly place and they can be connected to it, or whether they feel the universe is an unfriendly place and have a hostile relationship with life."

Among her various research and teaching activities, Dr. Borysenko conducts workshops for women with a variety of health concerns. The focus of these sessions, she says, is healing:

People blame themselves for not feeling well, and secondly blame themselves again if they clear up their relationship, practice forgiveness, change their diet, medicate, and their symptoms progress. I like to deal with that and the realization that your psychological health is certainly bearing on your physical health, but that healing is very different from curing and you can heal your life and die anyhow, which all of us will.

I think that the worst thing for women or men when they are using mind/body techniques to try to cure themselves physically is that too often they make their body and the status of their health the battleground. A lot of what we do is just dealing with healing in a general way, the sacredness of that, and with the idea that when we're in a state when we're aware that death isn't abstract but is something that may apply physically to us in the near future, it really helps you live your life more in the moment, and that is what healing is about anyhow. I like to help shift people away from the preoccupation with the body, which creates stress, to a preoccupation with living life with joy, which creates health.

A Few Mind/Body Techniques to Consider

Biofeedback Training

One of the leading mind/body therapies is biofeedback, in which an individual learns to consciously regulate bodily functions. Brain wave activity, cardiovascular and respiratory function, and skin temperature can all be influenced through biofeedback. In so doing, it is possible to relieve tension headaches, hypertension, incontinence, and other conditions.

Breathing Exercises

Slow, conscious, diaphragmatic breathing is a powerful tool for promoting relaxation and awareness.

Guided Imagery

Guided imagery uses the power of the mind to evoke a positive physical response. Studies have shown that it can decrease chronic nightmares, reduce substance abuse, and alleviate many other psychological and physiological problems.

Hypnotherapy

Hypnotic techniques can combat alcoholism, substance abuse, and overeating, as well as stress, sleeping disorders, and various mental health problems.

Meditation

This ancient practice has been proven to help alleviate hypertension and heart disease, along with stress, pain, and various other conditions.

Give Yoga a Chance

Yoga, qigong, and tai chi may be unfamiliar terms to you, but for millions of people across America they're becoming household words—and activities. These practices are as ancient as they are beneficial. Part of what's beneficial is that they're more meditative than fast-moving workouts. They generally employ very slow, methodic, and gentle movements, as well as a focus on breathing and consciousness.

Each of these techniques contains at least a three-pronged approach to health: improved muscle flexibility, strength, and tone; proper breathing; and relaxation, which may include creative visualization or other closed-eye exercises. This may sound strange, but keep your mind open. Studies show they're good medicine for women experiencing perimenopause. In fact, Dean Ornish, M.D., author of *Dr. Dean Ornish's Program for Reversing Heart Disease*, utilizes and recommends yoga to help people prevent or reverse heart disease and other illness. Furthermore, hospitals around the country have now integrated yoga into their programs for treating chronic pain, stress-related medical disorders, and anxiety disorders.

Yoga is likely the most accessible mind/body exercise, so it is profiled in this chapter. Additionally, most women find it to be an enjoyable way to integrate mind/body medicine into their lives. Yoga classes are offered through yoga centers, hospitals, gyms, dance studios, and colleges, or by private instruction. There are books and videotapes with detailed instruction that you can do at home. Like the other disciplines, yoga addresses the whole person and can be of help to people with a broad range of medical problems. The word itself is Sanskrit and means "to unite, to make whole." It's an excellent way to balance body, mind, and spirit.

Stretching is an integral part of what makes up yoga. But the stretches you'll do in these classes go beyond what you've ever done before—not in terms of stressing the muscles but by taking on postures or positions that stretch several muscles at once. According to the philosophy behind yoga, these positions open up the lines of energy that flow through the body, thus enabling more energy to blocked areas. The theory is that when energy flows to those areas, there's a greater opportunity for healing and body awareness. Whether there's scientific fact to back this up or not, it's almost certain you'll experience greater movement, strength, and inner peace if you utilize this wonderful approach to health.

These slow, deliberate stretches, and the proper breathing

that you'll learn while doing them, can be done at your own individual pace. You get to take yourself to the limits of your own body without stressing or straining yourself. Of course, you might be seated next to someone who can touch her nose to her knees without any difficulty. But that doesn't matter. That's her flexibility, not yours. The great news about yoga is that it will help everyone at any level of strength or flexibility. As long as you don't push yourself too hard, or set up rules of competition within your own head, you can reap the benefits of this wonderful exercise no matter what shape you're in.

Proof Positive of the Benefits of Yoga

Suza Francina is a certified Iyengar yoga instructor with more than 20 years of experience in the field of yoga and exercise therapy, as well as the director of the Ojai Yoga Center in Ojai, California, and has seen many cases of improved health and well-being of women who have begun to do yoga after a period of nonexercise. "People who attend yoga classes regularly for at least 6 months report that their increased strength and range of movement enables them to see life in an entirely different way," says Suza. "For some, that means they can return to other physical activities they thought they had lost forever: gardening, climbing stairs or up a hill, biking, dancing, reaching and bending without strain, being able to sit on the floor in various positions, and getting up and off the floor with confidence. For others it's simply realizing a new level of flexibility and fitness."

The Movements

Think about the way your body works, then use each joint in its most stable and functional anatomical plane. Avoid extending your limbs abruptly or in unnatural directions. Also, be careful not to hold a single position for too long. There is no set answer to the perennial question, "How long should I stay in the pose?" Long enough so that a healthy change has been made. Not so long that your body feels unhealthy strain or stiffens. Avoid mechanical repetitions and counting while exercising. Watch the flow of your breath and your body's response to a particular pose or exercise. Learn to tune into what your body is telling you.

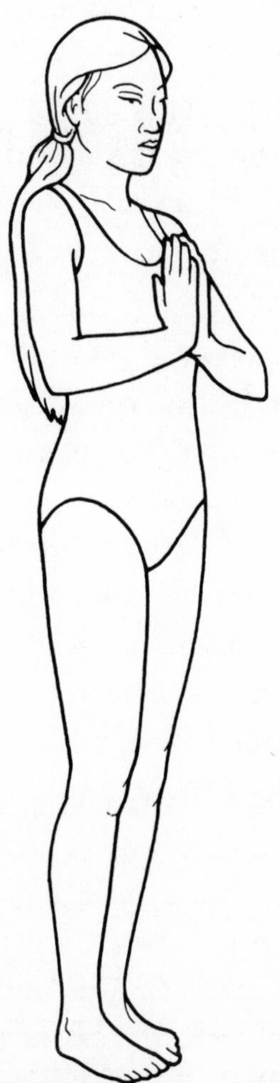

Namaste

Namaste (prayer) Position

Sit or stand and press your palms together in prayer position. This position helps to stretch the muscles in the hands and straighten the fingers. If your wrists hurt or you have carpal tunnel syndrome, practice Namaste with forearms touching.

- Gently press the palms and fingers of both hands together. As you breathe smoothly and evenly, encourage the fingers to move toward the thumb side of the hand. Hold for several breaths. Release the pressure, but keep the hands together for a few more breaths. Then repeat the effort three or four times.
- Gently, firmly, and evenly press the palms together. Smoothly open the fingers and spread them as wide as possible. Try to spread them evenly, moving them more and more toward the thumb side of the hand. Hold and stretch for a few breaths. Release and repeat.
- Firmly and evenly press the palms together, especially the parts of the palm at the base of each finger. Stretch the fingers backward, away from each other, gradually increasing the V-shaped space between them. Again, encourage the fingers to move toward the thumb side of your hands. Encourage your fingers to stretch for three or four more breaths. Release and repeat three or four more times.

Shoulder Stretch Practice

To avoid pulled muscles, overstretching, and joint strain, never force or rush your body into a yoga position. Use straps and belts to help you achieve a healthier, more balanced stretch.

If you cannot clasp your hands together, use a strap as a bridge between your two hands. This shoulder rotator exercise is one of the most basic corrective poses for removing stiffness from the shoulder joints.

- Stand (or sit) in your best, tallest posture. Pause for a moment to observe your breath. Allow yourself to smile. This will naturally relax your jaw and face muscles.
- Stretch your right arm straight up over your head and then bend your elbow so that your palm touches your back between the shoulder blades. Reach across with your left hand to move your elbow closer to your head.
- Release your left hand from your right elbow and bring your left arm straight back behind your body. Bend the left elbow, placing your hand in the middle of your back above your waist, palm out. Without distorting your posture or straining, try to clasp your hands together.
- If your fingers just barely touch, or if there is a big space between your hands, hold a strap or sock in your right hand and gradually work your hands together. Stretch up through the top elbow and down through the bottom elbow. Keep your head centered, face relaxed. Hold at least half a minute. Repeat on the right side. Lean from your more flexible side and repeat or hold longer on the tighter side.

Triangle Pose at Wall

- Make sure you have at least 6 feet of empty wall space. To improve posture, spend a few minutes every day standing tall with your back against the wall. If you tend to stoop forward, stretch your shoulders back and stand against the wall several times a day.
- Stand tall with your posture open, shoulders relaxed away from your ears, near the wall. Move your feet about 3½ to 4 feet apart (depending on the length of your legs), keeping your feet in line, facing forward, heels close to the wall.
- Breathe normally. Anchor and root your feet to the earth by pressing the soles of your feet deep into the floor.

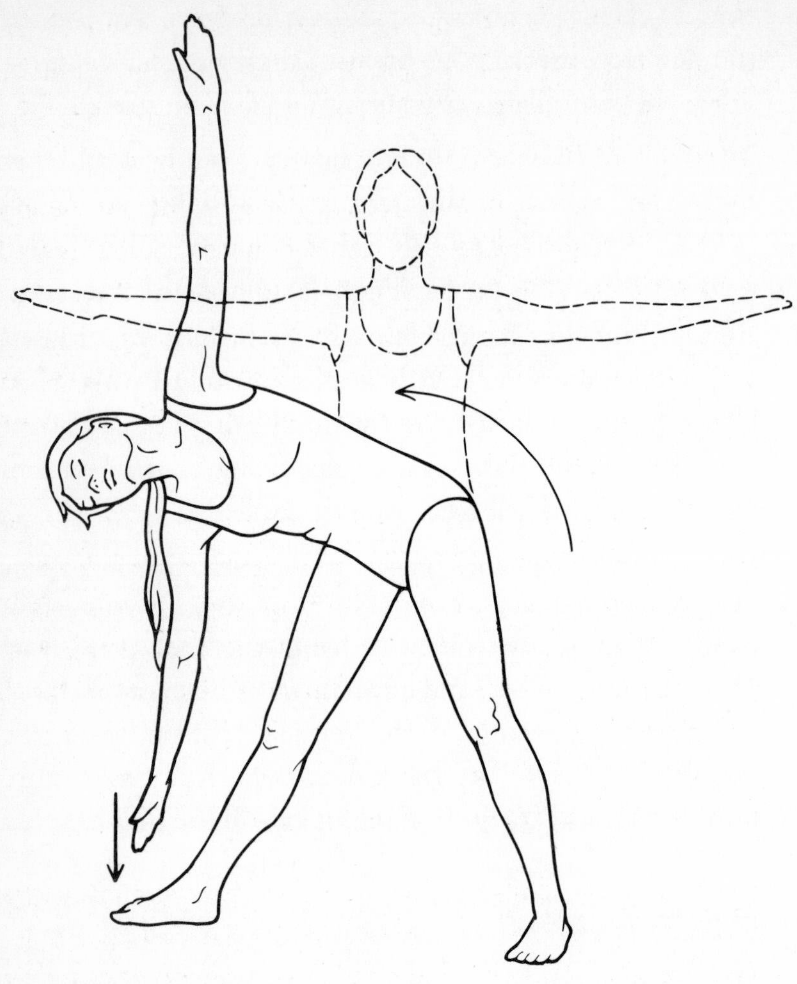

Triangle Pose

Activate your legs by pulling up the thigh muscles. Allow your body to become taller and taller, lengthening your spine upward. Raise your arms to shoulder level, palms facing down, and stretch out through your fingertips. Feel the center of your body expand and open.

- When you feel stable and centered in this position, turn the left foot about 15 degrees in, and the right foot 90 degrees out. Line up the right heel directly in line with the center of the left arch.
- Inhale, and on exhalation, stretch to the right from the hip joint so that your torso bends sideways as a unit toward your right leg. In the beginning, you may need to place your right hand on your leg or a chair. Extend your left arm up in line with the right arm, palm facing forward. If you feel unusual strain in your shoulder, try placing your left hand on your hip.
- Stay in the pose for several breaths, keeping your legs active, shoulders and neck relaxed. Come out of the pose on an inhalation, keeping your body close to the wall. Turn your feet to face forward. Relax back into the wall and pause for a moment to feel the effects of the pose. Repeat on the other side.

Downward Facing Dog Pose from the Floor

- Kneel on all fours on a nonslippery floor so that your hands do not slide. Position your knees slightly behind your hips, toes curled under, your feet and knees hip width (about 18 inches apart). Place your hands slightly in front of your shoulders, shoulder distance apart. Spread all 10 fingers wide apart and press both hands down onto the floor.
- On an exhale, straighten your knees and lift your bottom toward the ceiling so that your body forms a high upside-down V or pyramid shape. Raise your heels high off the floor and try to lift your bottom higher and higher. Press your hands deep into the floor as if you are pushing the floor away from you. After stretching for a few breaths with your heels lifted, try pressing your heels down toward the floor.

Step 1

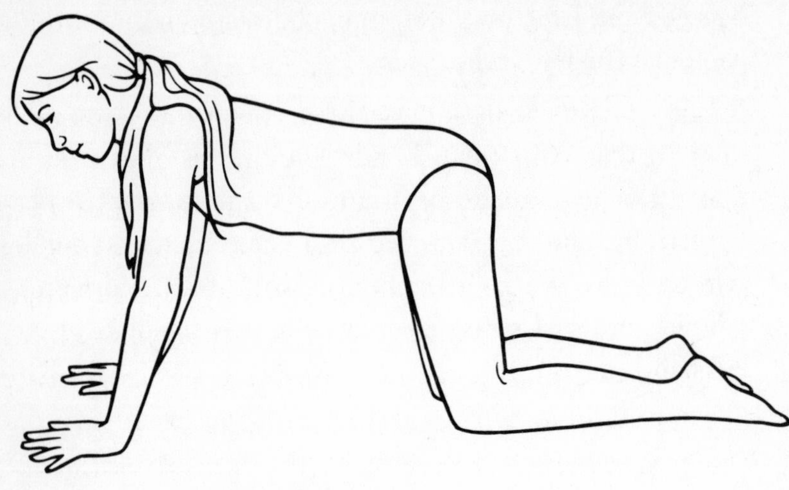

Steps 2 and 3

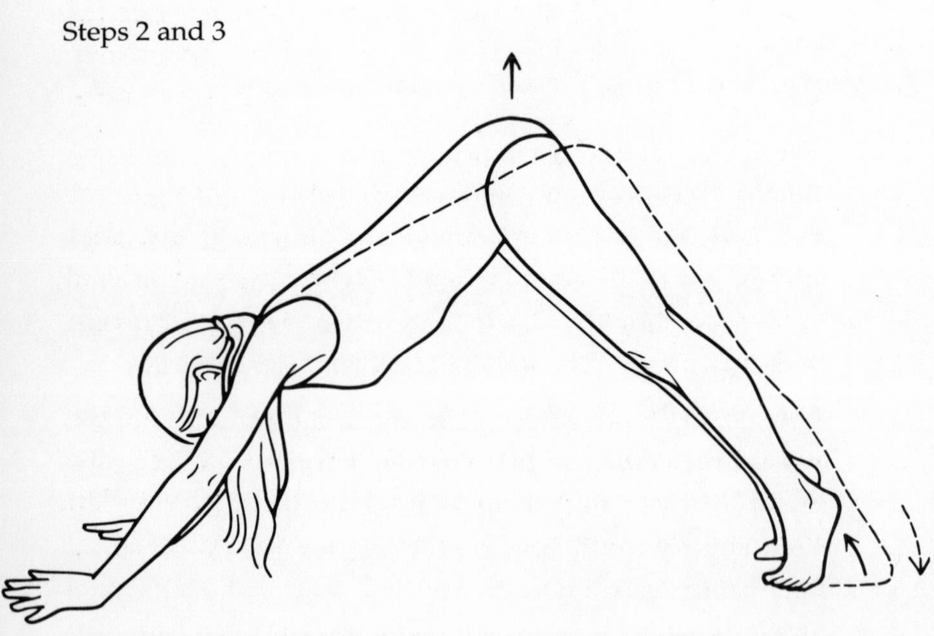

Downward Facing Dog

- Breathe smoothly, naturally. Keep your face and neck relaxed and soft. Imagine roots pulling your hands and feet into the earth while the top of your buttocks, your tailbone, extends toward the sky. Release and return to kneeling on all fours. Slowly lower your bottom back toward your heels and lower your torso and forehead to the floor.

A common complaint in this pose is pressure on the wrists. If your wrists are extremely sensitive, place a folded yoga mat (or folded blanket on the yoga mat to keep it from slipping) under the heel of your hands so that the wrist part of your hand is slightly elevated and supported by the extra cushioning. Do not stay in the pose if your back hurts, if you feel unusual pressure in the head or dizziness, or if your wrists and shoulders ache.

Lying-Down Leg Stretch with a Strap

A strap, towel, or soft belt around your feet while lying on the floor helps your spine to remain long and stable. Using a strap allows you to gradually stretch and lengthen stiff leg muscles without straining your back.

- Lie on your back with your knees bent, feet flat on the floor. If your head tilts back with your chin higher than your forehead, place a folded blanket under your head and neck. Check to see that your upper body is in line with your legs. Allow your back to relax into the floor.
- Bend your right knee in toward your chest and wrap a strap, towel, soft belt, or necktie around the ball of your foot. Hold the strap with your right hand. Stretch your left arm out in line with your shoulder on the floor, palm facing up.
- Slowly straighten your right leg and stretch your toes toward your face. Walk your hand higher up the strap

toward your foot until your arm is straight. Keep your shoulders and the rest of your back relaxed on the floor.

- If your right hand is quite far away from your foot, keep your left knee bent. If you find it easy to hold your big toe, or if your right hand is high up the strap close to your foot, you can deepen the stretch by practicing this pose with the bottom leg straight, extending through both heels. Stretch your toes toward your face to lengthen your calves and Achilles tendons.
- Smile and allow your face muscles to relax. Let your breath flow freely, stretching deeper as you exhale. Hold the strap firmly without creating tension in your hand. Enjoy the feeling of the back of your leg lengthening. Hold for about half a minute, longer as you learn to relax and cooperate with the pose. Repeat on the opposite side. If you are practicing with both legs straight, it is helpful to extend the lower heel into the wall.

As always, approach yoga with an awareness of your own needs and limitations, and monitor your progress daily. If your body feels better after you do it, you probably did it right. If it feels bad, maybe you overdid it or used a pose incorrectly. Ask for help. Talk with a qualified instructor or a physical therapist who knows about yoga techniques and get to the root of the problem before it gets to you.

Qigong and tai chi are other popular mind/body methodologies that could be beneficial. The best way to learn these techniques is by taking classes, which are commonly taught at health clubs and community centers as well as yoga studios. There are also books and videos available that will help you learn them at home.

CHAPTER TEN

Putting It All Together

You now have a pretty good idea of what is happening to your body and what you can do to manage your symptoms. It's up to you to create your personalized plan.

Once you've taken steps to balance your life and find a doctor who will be your partner in this program, you're ready to get started with your individualized plan. As you've seen, it's easier to do than you might have originally imagined. And you understand that it takes time. In fact, it may take you months to experiment, adding what works and subtracting the things that don't. That's why it's so important to keep a journal. Not only will it be your most loyal companion during this process, but it'll help you remember the highs and lows you experience.

A Case Study

Barbara, 37 years old, began experiencing perimenopause as a series of irregular periods. Some were heavier, others were lighter, and some months she wouldn't have a period at all. This, combined with a heightened sense of anxiety, despite the fact that family and career issues were stable for the first time in many years, led Barbara to consult with her physician.

Indeed, Barbara was experiencing perimenopause. In addition to her initial symptoms, she also had insomnia. As an entrepreneur and the mother of a preteen daughter, these symptoms were getting in the way, so Barbara designed her own perimenopause plan based on the steps described in this book. Here's a brief overview.

Step 1: Cleanse Your Liver

Barbara took part in a weeklong juice fast, followed by a slow introduction of foods to test for food allergies and intolerances. Barbara found that she was allergic to corn (a common allergy) and eliminated all forms of corn products from her diet.

Step 2: Use Natural Progesterone

Using the standard topical formula for beginning users of ⅛ teaspoon of natural progesterone twice daily, Barbara's periods regulated within 2 months. She now uses a maintenance dose of ⅛ teaspoon 4 days a week, 3 weeks out of every month.

Step 3: Follow Dietary Recommendations

Barbara was already feeding her family a good diet, but she made some changes to incorporate a greater variety of fresh vegetables and fruits, as well as substituting vegetarian protein foods, including tofu, for the meat she was serving at every dinner menu.

Step 4: Use Nutritional and Herbal Supplements to Balance Your Body and Reverse Symptoms

Barbara doubled her intake of B vitamins and began supplementing with 3000 milligrams of vitamin C, taken 6 times a day in 500-milligram intervals. She also began to take a tincture of black cohosh to balance her hormone levels.

Step 5: Exercise!

Work with the chart on page 188.

Step 6: Use Mind/Body Medicine

Work with the chart on page 188.

Barbara laid her plan out using a chart like this one. Find one that works for you.

Close Your Eyes and See

Now that you've charted out your next steps, guess what you get to do? That's right. You get to do what's on your chart. Here's a reminder of what your new life will bring:

- Some or complete relief from your symptoms
- Improved posture and appearance
- Heightened libido and better sex life
- Weight maintenance
- Feelings of vitality, joy, and appreciation for life
- Better circulation and digestion
- A healthier heart and reduced risk of heart disease and stroke
- Lower blood pressure
- Increased strength and stamina
- A sense of control over both pain and life

Exercise and Meditation Schedule

Barbara's Exercise and Meditation Schedule	*Monday*	*Tuesday*	*Wednesday*	*Thursday*	*Friday*	*Saturday*	*Sunday*
Meditate		X		X		X	
Yoga		X		X		X	
Stretching		X		X		X	
Walking with Daughter			X				

- A boost to the immune system, which means fewer colds, flu, and other common illnesses including cancer
- Improved relationship with yourself

Looking at the goals you've written down on paper can often seem overwhelming. Yet once you begin to tackle this program and see (and feel) some relief from your symptoms, the future will appear less daunting. Remember that this plan you've designed is creating a brand new foundation for your health—a foundation that you will build on for increased good health throughout your life.

The perimenopause transition is one of many you will experience throughout your life. In the time leading up to menopause, you have an opportunity to strengthen your body and prepare your mind to hurdle that next obstacle with confidence. Use this book as your guide and remember that no one has greater influence over your health than you do.

Glossary

adrenal glands small pyramid-shaped glands situated on top of each kidney that secrete various substances, among which are the steroid hormones androgen, estrogen, and progesterone.

amenorrhea failure to menstruate.

amino acid organic compound of carbon, hydrogen, oxygen, and nitrogen: the "building blocks" of protein.

antioxidant substance that prevents oxidation or inhibits reactions promoted by oxygen.

basal metabolic rate (BMR) temperature of the body at the time of awakening each morning.

bioflavonoid constituent of the vitamin C complex.

blood-sugar level amount of glucose (sugar) circulating in the bloodstream.

calcium balance net processes in which calcium enters the body through the diet and leaves the body through sweat, urine, and feces.

cervix narrow lower end of the uterus that extends into the vagina.

collagen protein that is the supportive component of bone, connective tissue, cartilage, and skin.

corpus luteum "yellow body" seen in the ovary after ovulation, the cells of which produce progesterone and estrogen as well as other hormones.

dysmenorrhea painful or difficult menstruation.

endocrine glands glands that manufacture hormones and release them into the bloodstream (such as adrenal glands, ovaries, and pancreas).

enzyme protein capable of producing or accelerating a specific biochemical reaction at body temperature.

estrogen female hormone responsible for stimulating the development of female secondary sex characteristics.

fibroids fibrous, noncancerous growths most commonly found in or on the uterus.

free radicals highly reactive molecular fragments, generally harmful to the body.

gamma-linolenic acid (GLA) polyunsaturated fat that is used by the body to produce certain prostaglandins that control several important body processes.

glucose simple sugar that is the usual form in which the carbohydrate exists in the bloodstream.

glycogen principal form in which a carbohydrate is stored in the body for ready conversion into energy; found in the liver in muscle tissue in particular.

hormone chemical substance produced in one part of the body and carried in the blood to another part of the body, where it has specific effects.

hysterectomy surgical removal of the uterus (a radical hysterectomy includes removal of the uterus, cervix, ovaries, egg tubes, and sometimes lymph nodes near the ovaries).

leuteinizing hormone (LH) hormone produced by the pituitary (a large surge of this hormone in each menstrual cycle precedes ovulation by 12 to 24 hours).

menarch beginning of menstruation.

metabolism sum of chemical changes; the building up or destruction of cells that takes place in the body.

neurotransmitter substance that transmits nerve impulses across a synapse; brain chemicals that are involved in carrying messages to and from the brain.

ovary one of two female organs containing the eggs and the cells that produce the female hormones estrogen and progesterone.

ovulation process during which a mature egg is released from the ovary.

oxidation process of combining with oxygen.

pancreas large glandular organ that extends across the upper abdomen close to the liver and secretes digestive juices into the intestinal tract; these juices contain enzymes that act upon protein, fat, and carbohydrates. Also secretes the hormone insulin directly into the blood.

pituitary gland small oval organ at the base of the brain that produces many important hormones (particularly follicle-stimulating hormone and leuteinizing hormone) and has been called "the master gland."

progesterone a steroid hormone responsible for the changes in the endometrium in the second half of the menstrual cycle preparatory for implantation, development of the maternal placenta, and development of the mammary glands. Used to treat menstrual disorders, among other problems.

prostaglandins one of several compounds formed from essential fatty acids and whose activities affect the nervous, circulatory, and reproductive systems and metabolism. Research indicates that a type of prostaglandin is implicated in muscular contractions and menstrual cramps.

serotonin substance present in many tissues (especially the blood and nerve tissue) that stimulates a variety of smooth muscles and nerves and is believed to function as a neurotransmitter.

thyroid gland organ at the base of the neck primarily responsible for regulating the rate of metabolism.

uterus complex female organ composed of smooth muscle and glandular lining; the womb.

vagina muscular canal in the female that extends from the vulva to the cervix.

vulva external female sex organ, composed of the major and minor lips (labia major and minora), the clitoris, and the opening of the vagina.

Sources

All About Eve: The Complete Guide to Women's Health and Well-Being. Tracy Chutorian Semler. New York: HarperCollins Publishers, 1995.

Alternative Medicine Guide to Women's Health 1. Burton Goldberg and the editors of *Alternative Medicine*. Tiburon, CA: Future Medicine Publishing, 1998.

Before the Change: Taking Charge of Your Perimenopause. Ann Louise Gittleman. New York: HarperCollins, 1998.

Cooking with Rachel. Rachel Albert. Oroville, CA: George Ohsawa Macrobiotic Foundation, 1989.

Coping with Your Allergies. Natalie Golos and Francis Golbita. New York: Simon & Schuster, 1986.

Diet for a Poisoned Planet. David Steinman. New York: Ballantine Books, 1990.

Dr. Atkins' Vita-Nutrient Solution: Nature's Answer to Drugs. Robert C. Atkins. New York: Simon & Schuster, 1998.

Dr. Christiane Northrup's Health Wisdom for Women Newsletter. Potomac, MD. (301) 424-3700.

Dr. Dean Ornish's Program for Reversing Heart Disease. Dean Ornish. New York: Random House, 1990.

Earl Mindell's Supplement Bible. Earl Mindell. New York: Fireside, 1998.

Encyclopedia of Nutritional Supplements: The Essential Guide for Improving Your Health Naturally. Michael T. Murray. Rocklin, CA: Prima Publishing, 1996.

Fibroid Tumors and Endometriosis Self-Help Book. Susan Lark. Berkeley, CA: Celestial Arts, 1995.

The Fountain of Age. Betty Friedan. New York: Simon & Schuster, 1993.

The Gynecological Sourcebook. Sara Rosenthal. Los Angeles: Lowell House, 1994.

Healing Mind, Healthy Woman: Using the Mind-Body Connection to Manage Stress and Take Control of Your Life. Alice D. Domar and Henry Dreher. New York: Henry Holt and Company, 1996.

Healing Visualizations. Gerald Epstein. New York: Bantam Books, 1989.

In Full Flower: Aging Women, Power and Sexuality. Lois W. Banner. New York: Vintage Books, 1993.

Kundalini Yoga: The Flow of Eternal Power. Shakti Parwha Kaur Khalsa. New York: Time Capsule Books, 1996.

Minding the Body, Mending the Mind. Joan Borysenko. New York: Bantam Books, 1987.

Natural Healing for Women: Caring for Yourself with Herbs, Homeopathy and Essential Oils. Susan Curtis and Romy Fraser. New York: HarperCollins, 1992.

Natural Progesterone, the Multiple Roles of a Remarkable Hormone. John R. Lee. Sebastopol, CA: BLL Publishing.

The Natural Remedy Book for Women. Diane Stein. Berkeley, CA: Crossing Press, 1992.

A New Prescription for Women's Health: Getting the Best Medical Care in a Man's World. Bernadine Healy. New York: Viking, 1995.

Nutritional Influences on Illness. Melvyn Werbach. Tarzana, CA: Third Line Press, 1996.

Ourselves, Growing Older: Women Aging with Knowledge and Power. Paula B. Doress-Worters and Diana Laskin Siegal. New York: Simon & Schuster, 1994.

Perfect Health. Deepak Chopra, M.D. New York: Harmony Books, 1990.

Recipes for Change: Gourmet Wholefood Cooking for Menopause. Lissa De Angelis and Molly Siple. New York: Dutton, 1997.

Relax and Renew: Restful Yoga for Stressful Times. Judith Lasater. Berkeley, CA: Rodmell Press, 1995.

SOS for PMS. Lissa De Angelis and Molly Siple. New York: Plume, 1999.

Spontaneous Healing. Andrew Weil. New York: Alfred A. Knopf, 1995.

Staying Healthy with Nutrition. Elson Haas, M.D. Berkeley, CA: Celestial Arts, 1992.

Still Life with Menu. Mollie Katzen. Berkeley, CA: Ten Speed Press, 1988.

What Your Doctor May Not Tell You about Premenopause, 1st ed. John R. Lee and Jesse Hanley with Virginia Hopkins. New York: Warner Books, 1999.

What Your Doctor May Not Tell You about Menopause, 2nd ed. John R. Lee with Virginia Hopkins. New York: Warner Books, 1997.

Wherever You Go There You Are: Mindfulness Meditation in Everyday Life. John Kabat-Zinn. New York: Hyperion, 1994.

The Whole Food Bible. Chris Kilham. Rochester, VT: Healing Arts Press, 1997.

Woman Heal Thyself: An Ancient Healing System for Contemporary Women. Jeanne Elizabeth Blum. Boston: Charles E. Tuttle Co., 1995.

The Woman's Encyclopedia of Natural Healing. Gary Null. New York: Seven Stories Press, 1996.

Women's Bodies, Women's Wisdom, 2nd ed. Christiane Northrup. New York: Bantam, 1998.

Women's Encyclopedia of Natural Medicine. Tori Hudson. Los Angeles: Keats Publishing, 1999.

Women's Health Companion, Self-Help Nutrition Guide and Cookbook. Susan M. Lark, M.D. Berkeley, CA: Celestial Arts Publishing, 1995.

Your Ideal Supplement Plan in 3 Easy Steps: The Essential Guide to Choosing the Herbs, Vitamins, and Minerals That Are Right for You. Deborah Mitchell. New York: Dell Publishing, 2000.

Resources

Videos

Living Yoga Practice Series

Quick yet well-balanced workouts designed to get specific results.

Moving to Mozart: Classic Exercise for an Ageless Body

This exercise video takes you through a set of stretching exercises set to music from Mozart's masterpieces. It includes introductory and secondary exercises for relaxation, alignment, strength building, and body proportioning.

The Physical Mind Workout

The latest in mind/body workouts is based on the world-famous Pilates method. Named for its creator, Joseph Pilates, this revolutionary toning and conditioning system stretches, strengthens, and realigns overworked joints and muscles.

Sources for Natural Progesterone Cream

AIM International, Inc.
3904 E. Flamingo Ave.
Nampa, ID 83687
(208) 465-5116
Distributor of Renewed Balance progesterone cream

Broadmoore Labs Inc.
3875 Telegraph Rd. #294
Ventura, CA 93003
(800) 822-3712
Maker of Natra-Gest and DermaGest progesterone creams

The Health and Science Research Institute
141 Glover Lane
Crawfordville, FL 32327
(800) 222-1415
www.health-science.com
Makers of Serenity for Women progesterone cream

International Health
8704 E. Mulberry St.
Scottsdale, AZ 85251
(602) 874-1419
(800) 481-9987
Distributor of Ess-Pro 7 natural progesterone cream

Life-flo Health Care Products
8146 N. 23rd Ave., Suite E
Phoenix, AZ 85021
(888) 999-7440
care@life-flo.com
Maker of Progestacare progesterone cream

Products of Nature
54 Danbury Rd.
Ridgefield, CT 06877
(800) 665-5952
Maker of Natural Woman progesterone cream

Transitions for Health, Inc.
621 SW Alder, Suite 900
Portland, OR 97205-3627
(503) 226-1010 or (800) 648-8211
Maker of Pro-Gest progesterone cream

Sources for Organically Grown, Hormone-Free, and Nitrite-Free Meat and Poultry

Food Outlets

Coleman Natural Beef is available at supermarkets throughout the United States including Grand Union stores in the New York City area, Purity Supreme in New England, A&P in New York and New Jersey, Bread & Circus in the Boston area, Big Y Foods in Massachusetts, and Farmer Jack stores in the Detroit, Michigan, area.

Foster Farms poultry is available in most supermarkets throughout the western United States. It has a rigorous pesticide residue elimination program, screening all shipments of grain. Subtherapeutic doses of antibiotics and other drugs are not used.

Holly Farms poultry is available throughout the eastern and midwestern states. It has a rigorous residue elimination program. Subtherapeutic doses of antibiotics and other drugs are not used. Holly Farms poultry is found in most supermarkets.

Kohler Farms of Wisconsin supplies hormone-free beef to supermarkets in Wisconsin and the Chicago area including Treasure Island. Look for the PURElean BEEF trademark.

Larsen Beef, produced without antibiotics or hormones, can be found in Kroger stores in Atlanta, Georgia, as well as King Kullen in Long Island, New York; Kash N Karry in the Tampa and Orlando, Florida, areas; and Dominicks in the Chicago area.

Laura's Lean Beef, produced without hormones, is available at Kroger stores in Kentucky and southern Indiana.

Maverick Ranch Lite Beef is produced without hormones or antibiotics and is lab tested for pesticide residues. It is available at King Supermarkets in Denver, Colorado; Schnucks in Saint Louis, Missouri; Kings Supermarkets in New Jersey; and Clemens in Philadelphia, Pennsylvania.

Organic Cattle Co. beef is certified organic and is available at supermarkets in the New York City area.

Quality Steaks produces hormone-free beef that is available at Star Markets in Massachusetts, First National Supermarkets in New England, and ABCO in the Phoenix, Arizona, area.

Associations

Center for Science in the Public Interest
Americans for Safe Food Project
1875 Connecticut Ave, NW, Suite 300
Washington, DC 20009-5728
(202) 332-9110, ext. 384

You can obtain a list of organic mail-order suppliers or hormone-free beef suppliers, both supermarket chains and mail-order home delivery, from this organization.

Eden Acres
Organic Network
12100 Lima Center Rd.
Clinton, MI 49236-9618
(517) 456-4288

Organic Network, a division of Eden Acres, offers a 150-page international directory or local statewide directories of suppliers of organic meats, poultry, fruits, and vegetables.

Associations

Educating yourself about healthier alternatives is the first step toward an improved diet. The following list tells you where to find a naturopathic physician, an organic food supplier, and more.

Complementary Healing

Acupressure Institute of America
1533 Shattuck Ave.
Berkeley, CA 94709
(510) 845-1059
(800) 442-2232

American Association of Acupuncture
and Oriental Medicine
433 Front St.
Catasauqua, PA 18032
(610) 266-1433

American Association of Naturopathic Physicians
601 Valley St., Suite 105
Seattle, WA 98109
(206) 298-0126
www.naturopathic.org

American Holistic Health Association
P.O. Box 17400
Anaheim, CA 92817-7400
(714) 779-6152
ahha@healthy.net

American Holistic Medical Association
4101 Lake Boone Trail
Raleigh, NC 27607
(919) 787-5181

American Massage Therapy Association
820 Davis St., Suite 100
Evanston, IL 60201-4444
(708) 864-0123

Doctor's Data, Inc.
P.O. Box 111
West Chicago, IL 60185
(800) 323-2784

For food allergy testing.

Holistic Health Directory and Resource Guide
42 Pleasant St.
Watertown, MA 02172
(617) 926-0200

Immuno Labs, Inc.
1620 West Oakland Park Blvd.
Fort Lauderdale, FL 33311
(800) 231-9197

This laboratory specializes in allergy and immunological testing.

Physicians for Social Responsibility
801 N. Farifax St., Suite 306
Alexandria, VA 22314
(703) 548-7790
(703) 548-7792
www.healthy.net/nch

World Chiropractic Alliance
2950 N. Dobson Rd.
Chandler, AZ 85224
(800) 347-1011

World Research Foundation
20501 Ventura Blvd., Suite 100
Woodland Hills, CA 91364
(818) 999-5483
(818) 227-6484 (fax)

Environmentally Friendly Foods and Products

Clean Water Action Project
1320 18th St. NW, Suite 300
Washington, DC 20036
(202) 547-1196

A lobbying group that seeks to protect the environment. They are especially concerned with water, waste, sewage, pollution, and wildlife.

Fighting Food Irradiation
Consumers United for Food Safety
P.O. Box 22928
Seattle, WA 98122
(206) 747-2659

Contact them to find out more about the irradiation of food. The organization's newsletter, *The Food Activist*, provides updates on national developments in food irradiation.

The Organic Foods Production Association
of North America
P.O. Box 1078
Greenfield, MA 01302
(413) 774-7511
(413) 774-6432 (fax)

Publications and memberships are available.

Pesticide Hotline
U.S. Environmental Protection Agency
NPTN Texas Tech University
Thompson Hall, Room S129
Lubbock, TX 79430
(800) 858-7378

A telephone hot line open Monday to Friday from 8 A.M. to 6 P.M. (EST) to answer questions on pesticides from the medical field, general public, and veterinarians.

Socially Responsible Shopping
Seeds of Change
621 Old Santa Fe Trail, Suite 10
Santa Fe, NM 87501
(505) 983-8956

An organic seed company that specializes in biodiversity. Their catalogue is available by mail or in some health food stores.

Vegetarian Journal
Vegetarian Resource Group
P.O. Box 1463
Baltimore, MD 21203
(410) 366-8343

A nonprofit vegetarian resource group whose main goal is to educate the public on health, nutrition, and the environment.

Vegetarian Times
1140 Lake St., Suite 500
Oak Park, IL 60301
(708) 848-8100

A glossy color magazine that offers recipes as well as informative articles and the latest news in vegetarian lifestyles.

Herbal Medicine

American Herbalists Guild
P.O. Box 1683
Soquel, CA 95073
(408) 464-2441

Herb Research Foundation
1007 Pearl St., Suite 200
Boulder, CO 80302
(303) 449-2265
www.herbs.org

Quality Life Herbs
P.O. Box 565
Yarmouth, ME 04096
(207) 842-4929
(207) 846-3168

Mind/Body Medicine

American Board of Hypnotherapy
16842 Von Karman Ave., Suite 475
Irvine, CA 92606
(800) 872-9996

Center for Mind/Body Medicine
5225 Connecticut Ave. NW, Suite 414
Washington, DC 20015
(202) 966-7338

Mind/Body Health Sciences, Inc.
393 Dixon Rd.
Boulder, CO 80302
(303) 440-8460

Mind/Body Medical Institute
Deaconess Hospital
1 Deaconess Rd.
Boston, MA 02215
(617) 632-9525

Nutritional Supplementation

American Academy of Nutrition
3408 Sausalito Dr.
Corona Del Mar, CA 92625
(800) 290-4226

American College of Nutrition
722 Robert E. Lee Dr.
Wilmington, NC 28480
(919) 452-1222

Consumer Nutrition Hotline
(800) 366-1655

Corsello Centers for Nutritional Complementary Medicine
200 W. 67th St.
New York, NY 10019
(212) 399-0222

National Institute of Nutritional Education
1010 S. Joliet St., #107
Aurora, CO 80012
(303) 340-2054

Price Pottenger Nutrition Foundation
P.O. Box 2614
La Mesa, CA 91943-2614
(619) 574-7763

Women's Health

Endometriosis Association
8585 N. 76th Place
Milwaukee, WI 53223
(800) 992-3636

Menstrual Health Foundation
Womankind
P.O. Box 1775
Sebastopol, CA 95473
(707) 522-8662

National Women's Health Network
(212) 593-2141

Planned Parenthood Federation of America
810 Seventh Ave.
New York, NY 10019
(212) 541-7800
www.plannedparenthood.org

Yoga

International Kundalini Yoga Teachers' Association
(505) 753-0423

Yoga Journal
2054 University Ave.
Berkeley, CA 94704

Yoga Research and Education Center
(707) 928-9898
www.yogaresearchcenter.org

Index